Alpha Book Publisher
www.alphapublisher.com
ISBN: 978-1-954297-66-1

Ordering Information:
Quantity sales. Special discounts are available on quantity purchases by corporations, associations, and others. For details, contact the publisher at the address above.
Orders by U.S. trade bookstores and wholesalers.
Visit www.alphapublisher.com/contact-us to learn more.

Printed in the United States of America

Table of Contents

WHO ARE YOU REALLY?

Did you ever think to yourself why do I feel this way or why am I down? Maybe you might say to yourself it will pass and yet the feeling and thoughts seem to linger day to day. The feeling is starting to become normal and you may say to yourself, "Is this supposed to be who or what I am?" Stop right there! Let me fill you in on something I wish someone would have told me. You are not your feelings and your thoughts. You just happen to be expressing those at the moment, however, you do not have to embody the belief that this is who you are. You, at this moment, may be saying to yourself, "Then why do I feel this way constantly? Why do I have these thoughts and how can you tell me about ME?" This book is not about telling you who you are but it will give insight into what you are dealing with. Let's begin shall we.

NEGATIVE STATE OF MIND

Listen, there will be no sugar coating from this point forward, what you are dealing with is negativity which leads to a negative mind set, negative actions and then a negative systematic automated process that finally becomes your state of being. This state of being brings the illusion that your thoughts are who you are, but really you are in your lower self. In this part of self, you experience all kinds of emotions like depression, anger, loss of will power, confusion, aggression, sadness, lack of self-esteem, lack of confidence, internal and external suffering, disempowerment and a host of other mind thoughts. Listen, it sucks, I know, but it really is a part of you and at this time in life this negative part of you has decided to rear its ugly head. Let me assure you that you are not the first to experience this nor will you be the last.

2

Negativity usually stems from when our ego feels threatened, vulnerable and unprotected. We experience negativity in small chunks throughout life, like your partner dumps you so you play sad breakup songs; the friend you once had deserted you so feel alone or somebody drinks the last of your juice that has your name on it for the umpteenth time and you want to snap their fingers...sorry I had a moment. These moments tend to pass and we go back to being our regular selves again until a shitstorm of overwhelming proportions gets thrown our way on a day to day nearly moment by moment basis. That is when it begins.

WHY ME???

Because you are the chosen one silly (if not you then who else?) Okay that was a bad joke, but that is exactly what life to you now feels like - a bad joke being played on you constantly as if you are being singled out and punked relentlessly. Now, here you go pointing the finger playing the blame game, saying it is everybody else's fault but your own. It may very well be other people who played a part in your downfall; however, you have to take responsibility and hold yourself accountable too. This thing that you are going through may not have started with you but it definitely ends with you. Do yourself a favor and own up to your part in this fast so you can get through this and move the hell on. It's not that easy, but it's a start. You have to confess to yourself that you had something to do with this. Take a minute and say "It is my fault I am in this mess" see now don't you feel better? This is the part where you scream and say "Hell No" well good, but at least you got it out. By admitting your part and taking ownership of it, you just earned my respect. You are now ready to move forward to understanding what you are experiencing.

Besides, if we don't know what we don't know, how can we do anything about it without understanding it first. Let us take a further look into what this condition is.

NEGATIVE ORIENTATION

You may be thinking that you did not show up to work for this crap. Of course, you didn't, but somehow it found you and now you are stuck in this state. Negative orientation is a state or condition in which one finds themselves that skews their perspective on self and everything around them, causing internal conflict to their psyche and external conflict to people, places and things surrounding them. Being in this condition also has a draining effect which causes those around you to become lowered in energy, offended, detached and dissociated. I know you have felt this before but you can't really see it or put your finger on it, but you can recall a time when this has happened to you. For example, one day your friend who normally is humorous and full of life walks past without saying hello or making a joke. Their head is down and they have this lost look on their face, as if they are looking for or questioning something going on. You go to say hello, but they say not now. You later catch up with them to ask what is going on but they say "leave me alone I am not in the mood".

You may say "well you can talk to me about anything" and before you can get it out, they yell "I don't need your help. You are annoying me and being nosey. Stay away from me". I am pretty sure that's because you care for your friend, you're now feeling pretty low and maybe confused or upset at the friend you were trying to help. This uneasy feeling may have started a projection of negative energy from the friend who is in negative orientation. This state is hard to understand if you have never experienced it and it causes you to question yourself and may even impose doubt into your life and personal identity.

We have been taught as children that life is our oyster and that we can be whatever we want to be. What we weren't warned about was the forces we could face within ourselves and how to deal with them in a mentally healthy way. We are also taught to be selfish and to seek everything outside of self and that these things will bring us fulfillment (e.g., Wait! Hello! What about ME?) My question is, "What about you?" This society does not care about you; but more about what you can do for it. You go through life not understanding and building that relationship with self; so, you then seek validation of your actions and identity from external sources. No wonder when you face adversity! You don't feel like you, because

6

you never thought that negative orientation would be a part of you in the first place. This part of you was always brushed off and never dealt with. Sayings like 'get over it', or 'nobody likes a crybaby', causes a person to snap out of it on the outside, while on the inside these feelings fester.

WHO ELSE DEALS WITH THIS?

Everybody is susceptible to dealing with a negative state of mind or conditioning. No one person or group is exempt. Negative energy is transferable. It is how we deal with this energy that either puts us in the driver seat giving us control or keeps us riding the passenger side causing it to control us; thus, causing self-inflicted pain or causing pain to others for the betterment of their ego.

Truth be told when one gives into negativity, it can be used to destroy oneself. Generally, we as humans have not been taught how to deal with such feelings and we mask it as if it is a disease and we don't talk about it. This is one of the worst things you can do seeing as being alone can cause volatile thoughts and behaviors to occur. Speaking to people who haven't dealt with it can also be detrimental because they have no experience with it and they are likely to ridicule, ostracize or shame you. Lastly, being with people who are familiar with this state, but use it in an unhealthy way, will most likely cause a person to go further down an unwanted path causing more emotional rifts in the psyche of one's mind.

Awareness of negative orientation increases the chances of one getting out of this state. But what if this state of being causes lack of awareness. Now, how should this be navigated properly without causing further harm to the one inflicted by this condition. You may have heard the phrase "to be aware is to be alive" however, it is not just concerning your external environment, but it also concerns your internal environn

with self in a healthier manner will allow access to an ei

acknowledge your negative thought(s) and then immedi

like to do is run with the thought of seeing where it m

proper questioning right then and there. If we learn to

begin to see if this thought is servicing us or not. For

thought? Will this thought better my mood or decreas

this thought bother me? What thought do I want to have besides this and how will I go about

changing my thought pattern?"

Objective questioning will help you to effectively deal with the negative thoughts while subjective questioning leaves an opening to go down a rabbit whole just to find no carrots there. It leaves room to interpret rather than knowing for certain why you may feel or think this way. You may be thinking that I don't talk to myself. That is crazy and I'm not crazy. Well, you need to learn to get a little crazy and not only talk to but also answer your own questions! This is the only way to build self-trust and keep healthy thought patterns is to have those crucial conversations with, you guessed it, yourself.

How can you start these conversations, if you are not comfortable with yourself inwardly? Hey, let's start by building some inner confidence. Here is a challenge for you, ask yourself what you don't like about you and answer yourself honestly. Next, ask yourself what do you like and never want to change about you? Then, ask yourself what could I improve about me? Please be candid; I am sure your conscience would appreciate that. Finally ask yourself did you learn something new about yourself? If so, then guess what you just built? Trust in yourself by being confidence, because you see your upside, downside, opportunities for increased self-awareness. Doing routine checks like this about different case your life will help you get to know you better and stay focused about what serves what does not. If you did not learn anything about yourself then the issue may be even ore severe than you realize.

If after questioning oneself, you find nothing was discovered or uncovered and things seem fine, chances are you were conditioned to be that way. See, the funny thing about being conditioned without realizing it is that these little glitches come up in your life and your thoughts may say this is normal, but your gut says something does not feel right. You at this point are not in the know about self. You have actually been programmed and even worse you may still be under this programming. Programming can be a good or bad thing depending on if it serves you in a healthy way or not. For example, if you were taught that eating fast food every night was perfectly normal, but then 5 years later you go to a doctor to find out you have been diagnosed with diabetes and obesity, chances are your program was not serving you well.

This would mean this program is no good and that rewiring must occur. A program must first be recognized before it can be updated or switched out. Once an update occurs, you can begin to then be served properly in a way that better suits you. If you find out a subscription was not providing you with what you wanted, would you cancel it? I am sure the answer is yes. So, what programs have you conformed to without knowing? Let us find out together.

NEGATIVE PROGRAMMING

YOU WERE BORN INTO THIS

The first couple of years that we enter into this world, mind programming begins! From mannerisms and tones, to speech and food choices and even being told to you what is good or bad. Who does this to you? It starts with your parents and then, as your world expands, to family, teachers, friends, doctors, religion, community, environment, television, radio, movies, marketing, advertising, etc. begin to influence who you should be. This, in the beginning, seems to cause no harm and is meant to show you the way of the world. However, over time, these influences can play pivotal parts in our lives and can have a lasting impact as well. Not all influences are meant to serve us; some are meant to serve others and you just so happen to be the one to fall for the shenanigans. Truthfully, you will come to find that if you just blindly follow external influence without having an internal compass, chances are you will become someone else and not who you want to be.

Have you ever driven down the highway and saw a billboard advertisement and thought I want that to be me or I want that for myself? Come on, sure you have, maybe a woman sees one with a guy proposing to a lady with a diamond ring outside a beautiful home smiling and here comes my favorite part. The advertisement tells you where you should go to get this ring and as a woman you start to think I want a man to take me there to get one and I'll be happy! Or as a guy, you see a billboard with a man in a nice suit about to get into the car that conveys high status. Right before he gets into the car he looks toward the camera with the squinty eye and a smirk as if he is living out his dream. As a guy, you think I got to have that car so I will be able to impress women and my co-workers in that. Hey! That woman may feel good for the first couple of months of having the ring and the guy may impress her with the car, but in reality, you were just programmed to think this would mean happiness for you. Fast forward, what if you fell on hard times and had to pawn the ring or that car gets taken by repossession? How happy are you then? How desperate are you to get back this thing that defined your happiness, self-image and identity? It is this type of programming that gets us the most because it sells us the possibility of what could be without the consequence of true reality.

Another example of this type of programming is let's say you were told to never talk to this person or group of people because they do not mean you any good. But then you see them walking past you down the street and they say hello. Do you keep your head down and walk past quickly or worse say don't speak to them at all? You have been programmed to fear something or someone whom you do not know. Another form of this type of programming: let's take the same case scenario and you do happen to say hello back and then that person tries to attack you. Now based on that experience, it reinforces your programming further not wanting to deal with anyone or group that looks like the culprit. Now you have bias in your future dealings with anyone who looks like this type of person. Again, you were programmed this time by your own subconscious and those programs are the hardest to reverse. These examples are just a few ways in which we can become slaves to external and internal forces especially when we lack self-awareness. Don't worry, we will talk about self-awareness later, so stay tuned.

Programming must have context because without it we take things at face value without even considering whether this is serving me or failing me. How many relationships could you have had or partnerships that could have been wonderful or freedoms you could have enjoyed or places you could have experienced, but you didn't all due to your limited beliefs from involuntary programming? This is what happens when the program has not given you context, it's just been given in bits and pieces. Now I am not saying go get to know or see and do everything to find context, because it does not work that way. First, you should ask yourself, is it even worth it to you? What does this mean to me? How will this build me up or tear me down? Why do I want to know about this person or thing? Questions like these will help you put certain things in context before even pursuing what you are going to do, which will give you clear understanding internally before seeking it externally. Basically, what I am saying is go within first to figure out if you really want to get that ring, that car, get to know that person, take that opportunity or travel to that specific place before outwardly starting the process of doing so.

We are so programmed to social norms that we are apprehensive about going inside ourselves first to acknowledge if self is okay with this. We just do as we are told because this is how it has always been done and doing anything else is uncivilized or shameful or risky or whatever! We must first question ourselves before we just fall in line with what is and has been going on without a second thought. Why do we constantly give of ourselves to something we can care less about, chase after possessions, deny those hobbies that interest us, but conform to what we dislike, shun relationships when secretly we want one just like it? Well, we all have been programmed.

THE RADIO BOX SELLS FEELINGS

Ah yes! The beloved radio where you get to hear the commentating from your favorite pastimes, listen to your favorite music genre and even hear the latest gossip on the rich and famous. Yeah! When you hear these things, it makes you feel like you are there and in the know of what is going on. Sound moves us and if we are not paying close attention, we then move to the rhythm without thinking or truly listening. These sound waves evoke feelings ranging from sadness and pain to joy and happiness. The funny thing is how can we go from feeling one way to another just by hearing something being broadcast. Well, it is because we, on a subconscious level already had implanted thoughts of what we were hearing based on teachings and experiences. Now if this is so, this should mean we can change our mood back to what it was before hearing what we heard. Whether intentional or unintentional once we attach a feeling to something it then is a monstrous challenge to overcome, because it feels real as if it is happening to us.

A feeling will bypass logic and go into abstraction very easily if we are not careful with our emotions. Once we get emotional, we tend to get caught up in what we are being told when truthfully what is being told to us does not directly impact us. This is not saying we can't get into our emotions when a situation calls for it, but rather we should not stay in that emotion especially if it's one that will debilitate or cause stress. The issue here is when we have been programmed to listen to the radio for the latest music, news, and entertainment we do not manage what is coming into our thought process and what is going out. This means we are not actively monitoring our behavioral responses to the broadcast; we now are operating on autopilot where all the fun stuff being fed to us gets to fill our subconscious brain. Days, weeks or months later we find ourselves acting out the feelings or repeating the words from what we heard prior to. We may even ask ourselves, "Where did that come from?" Look out my friend, that was an implanted thought.

TELEVISION TELLS US A VISION

Having a vision of your own is one thing but being told a vision is completely different. When you have a vision, it is you seeing the possibilities of your own dream. When a vision is being told and sold to you, a person can see only the possibilities from that specific thing being shown. This limits possibilities for oneself, because if repeatedly watched you can only see what is in front of you, not what is beyond you. When you watch a motion picture you see yourself in certain characters that you relate to or identify with. If one is not aware, they may pick a persona they want to be and attempt to act out that character, instead of taking time to get to know oneself. When we see our favorite movie or tv characters get what we think we want for ourselves, subconsciously we will try to get the same things.

I am not saying anything is wrong with watching shows on television and movies for entertainment. The issue is if we are wanting to live out our lives vicariously through specific characters. We choose to embody these characters based on what we have seen. When we use our imagination, we can create our own character to become not someone else's made up character. We create the vision of ourselves in its entirety. This allows us to be fully aware of what we want to become. Having a vision of our own gives us purpose, something to reach for, fulfillment, room for possibility and breathes life into us. What is being shown to us by the media is full of negative imagery. If we are not conscious of what we are consuming this can make us act in a way that can lead us to go against our own character. Television can be the greatest influence in potentially molding either positive or negative thinking. For example, consistently watching commercials may fill your head with subliminal messaging or selling you convenience.

Therefore, commercials are created to cleverly convince you to purchase a product or service to make your life easier, give you more value or save you time. Truth be told, if you don't know what is right for you then you are susceptible to buying these things and still feeling empty. That emptiness comes from feeling the high of purchasing something, but gradually the high comes down after you realize this is not quite what you thought it would be. When you know more about self and what self requires, you won't be so quick to consume in order to be fulfilled. You will consider what you are being shown and see it for what it is: a visual sales pitch, a projected thought or an idea being delivered. Once you understand you are being told a message or shown a vision, you then can choose whether you want to receive them or not. It would be fair warning to say before you accept somebody else's vision you should probably have one of your own.

THEY TRY TO PROTECT, INSTEAD THEY PROJECT

Does anyone have a relative, friend, teacher, parent or associate telling you what is best for you. They may say phrases like 'you should or shouldn't do this' or 'you are not good at that, do this instead' or 'that won't make you any money, get a real job'? I'm quite sure this sounds familiar. Unfortunately, they are just giving you advice based on their perception and life's experiences.

The issue here is that these people can play such a pivotal part in your life because what they say is usually taken to heart which may become discomforting and hurtful.

If you are not deeply rooted in self-awareness, you then become an involuntary victim to the limitations based on the advice of others. Listen, this is not to say that they don't' have good intentions or don't want the best for you because in most cases they do. They may be concerned so they think that they are just encouraging you to avoid as many pitfalls as possible or not to make mistakes based on their experiences. Here is a harsh truth! If you do not fail sometimes, you cannot learn. It's that simple, but yet, because of fear we try to avoid failing.

The fear comes from what we have been told repeatedly by the very people who play major roles in our development. If told long enough over time, like magic poof, it becomes real to us and fear comes from going against something we have been told is not good for us. I cannot tell you how many times I have personally gone through this or have witnessed people going through this. It is one of the worst things that can happen to a person. Here is why the very essence of your being is being conflicted due to the very fears and downfalls of others. Short version - their fear becomes your fear and if in low consciousness you will not be aware of this overtaking. As if we do not have our own personal inner battles to overcome, now we deal with lost battles of others being cast upon us. Either one of two things can happen, we overcome or succumb.

As a result, we will succumb because all the sources around us tend to push us towards giving up and going the easy route where it's safer and less dangerous. Listen, this is not encouraging you to set out to do something violent to yourself and others. This encourages you

17

to chase after your dreams and goals regardless of what others have done because this is your life to live and not theirs. Do yourself a favor and get around people who you see are doing something worthwhile. Be encouraged by their bold actions, work ethic and high energy. If you chose to stay around people on lower levels the higher a chance that you will stay on a lower level too. If you are scared to leave them behind, the good news is you can always come back. Go!

Take a chance on yourself for once and stop living for others. Will it suck for a while? Yes. Will you be scared? Yes. Will there be times of doubt? Yes. But in the end will you be better? Hell yes! I assure you that this will set you up not to have any regrets in the long run. Look! People will try to project negative energy onto you like baby vomit but your job is not to let it get on you. If there is someone you love or value telling you not to do something, extract the good out of what they are saying, but in the end follow what feels right for you, because only you know what is right.

YOU BELIEVE IN EVERYTHING BUT YOURSELF

You have been taught to believe everything outside of you. These beliefs can be very real for you and even guide you down a better path. As long as these beliefs serve you and do not endanger others, go for it! The issue in our society is that we are taught to believe in other things, but there is very little focus on belief in ourselves. We can be empowered by our beliefs but you must be one with your belief not separate from it. Walk in your faith! Practice what you preach! Become that which you believe! When you believe enough with conviction at a certain point you begin to know yourself. This belief now becomes your truth and you can't go wrong.

When we only have an external belief, when something goes wrong, we tend to blame that which we believe in and not ourselves. News flash! You played a major role in it too, so while you are pointing a finger at everyone else remember there are three pointing back at you. I always wanted to say that! (Smile) When we don't believe in ourselves, we do not take responsibility for our actions, therefore we blame something outside of ourselves and we use something like our belief as a cop out. Trust me, aligning with your beliefs will make life better for you, because it won't be a crutch, it will become a source of power. Listen, let me tell you something! YOU ARE ENOUGH! YOU MATTER! YOU ARE MEANT TO BE HERE! The question now becomes what are you going to do about it? You have every right to be yourself just as the next person. So, why do you have limited beliefs in yourself? Let's look at your internal world and the darkness that dwells within.

THE DARK SPACE

FALLING INTO THE DARKNESS

I don't find it easy writing this portion of the book. So, please bear with me as we expose some ugly truths about what we are made of and what we can turn into, if we do not take heed. Let me start by saying we are made of light and darkness. Yeah! That's right! We have both energies inside which are always in constant battle and one will eventually gain control over our vessel. When we consume love, it brings out the light just as hatred (when it is consumed) brings out the darkness. Before I continue, let me tell you that "I hate everyone equally!" Okay! That is a joke to try and make this chapter lighthearted. Though this saying may contain sarcasm, it also contains truth. Let me tell you why.

Love is on the same line as hate. They are just on opposite ends of the same emotional spectrum. Here is an example. Have you ever had someone you hated become your most beloved best friend? What about someone you love becoming your worst hated nightmare. Do you see what I am getting at? These states of being are two opposite sides of the same coin.

Our perception is just skewed due to what we have seen, heard and have been taught. These two things are not separate from one another in fact they are the same. If you play music and turn it up, it is called loud music. But if you turn it low then it is called low music and guess what? It is still just music playing. What is the temperature? Either hot or cold but it is still just temperature, right? I think you get the point I am making now. Let's move on. Depending on the state you are in you can go from one side to the other rather quickly throughout your day, week, or month. But it is when we go to the furthest parts where things start to change drastically.

The term "the fall" you may have heard of this, in movies, fictional books, and even biblical stories. The thing is that the fall is real. Imagine for a second that you don't care anymore, you don't feel content, you feel empty, pain, anger, sadness, confusion, resentment, rage, and fear daily. Welcome to a world of hate buddy! Since this elevator of yours came crashing down to the darkness, you now have to find a way back up to the light with no stairs, no ladder, no rope or climbing equipment to get you there. In these parts of yourself, you will face the demons that haunt you, fears that stagnate you and the devilish part of you that rules this realm of your being. You will come to find once you are here you cannot simply leave.

You can either do one of two things: fight for your life to get out or give in and accept this as fate. It is scary isn't it, but it is very real. Stop and think for a minute before further reading this. Ask yourself, 'have I almost gone to this dark space before? What did I do to stop before going all the way? What was my saving grace?' If you can figure this out now, then you will be ahead of the curve and prepared for when it comes time to face your own internal darkness. I personally have gone down this road and guess what guys, I made the choice at one point to give in and not fight. I just said this must be the way it is meant to be. I am not going to be able to turn this around, this must be my lot in life, to suffer.

The more I fight it the more it takes hold of me; I might as well do what this dark force inside wants me to do. I became a slave to negative thoughts, which lead to negative actions and ultimately a negative perception of life itself. My Ego was fully immersed in this way of being and it would take me on a ride I would never forget.

I HATE MYSELF

Why me?!!!! Why is this happening to me?! I hate this world. I hate the people in it. I hate everything about it and I hate myself! AHHHH!!! These thoughts would become my new norm. What did I do to deserve this? It's not my fault I am this way, it's because of him, her, and them. Why should I have to go through this while they all get away scot-free? They all make a joke of this as if this is a game, but this is my life. They don't understand the pain! I want them to feel what I feel, deal with the thoughts I deal with and suffer like I suffer! So, you don't care to listen, understand, and support? Then fine I don't need you. In fact, I will use you just like you use me! I long for the day you stop smiling because that is when I will laugh the hardest. (Ha! Ha! Ha!). Insert psycho villain here. Yeah, so that became my internal dialogue and how I viewed my external world.

Now in truth some people did have dealings in my downfall, but the most important person was, hello, myself! We have this little thing that makes a big impact called the power of choice. We can always choose and with that choice comes a consequence, whether positive or negative. We must learn to be responsible as much as we can with our choices.

People, if you have learned nothing else from the warnings I bring, note that if you stopped reading this book right now, that you have the power of choice. Now I did not understand this power at the time because I thought things were happening to me and that I was not given a choice in the matter. So, I went into full on victim mode. Now this has something to do with what I faced as a child and the light heartedness I carried back then, but we will get into that a little later so stick around. My hatred grew for myself, it seemed like the more I gave into the darkness internally the more I attracted darkness externally. Now in the dark is when the Ego is in full bloom, so I had some great instantly gratifying times during this period of my life, but in most cases, it left me emptier than I was before. See ladies and gents, I was seriously in a very low state of awareness; so, at this point, I acted purely out of scarcity and fear of the unknown. I had consciously lost control of myself. Well, if that was the case then who was in the driver seat? Answer, my shadow self, you know the one who cares about nothing but self. Listen, wake up!

This may sound like some great fictional tale, but this is what we all must come face to face with sooner or later. Continue to be naïve if you want but that which you are not aware of has the upper hand and the element of surprise. While you are waiting like a sitting duck that is when you will be captured and hurled into "the fall" with the light slowly dimming, the further you go down. When you awake from your fall, you will open your eyes to nothingness.

IN THE DARKEST SPACE YOU WILL FIND NO LIGHT THERE

Here lies the creepiest, scariest, and ugliest part of self. Welcome to your own personal hell if you will. It is here that you will know what true torture feels like. Where physical torture lasts a moment in time, mental and spiritual torture lasts all day every day without fail. At times it can be very intense and at other times be very subtle. You are now a wanderer in your own darkness desperate to find the light again, but not worth enough for the light to shine upon you. You are sunken down in the depths of self, most thoughts are terrifyingly negative and even positive moments in life you cannot appreciate.

Welcome to the "Dark Space" I coined the term myself especially since I went on an unwanted vacation there. This Space has a vast amount of tests and trials to overcome and many lessons to learn from. Here you will find no relief, no refuge, no comfort, no compassion, no empathy, no purpose, no self-respect, no strength, and no end to it all - just pain. I think I painted the picture well enough for you. Here is the deal, this is your new home so get used to it because it only gets better from here. Speaking from experience I never really felt lonely or understood loneliness fully until I fell into this place. I felt people would never understand, I acted as if all was okay but deep down, I knew I was withering away. The void in my life kept getting bigger and bigger. The bigger it got the more stuff I tried to fill it with such as partying, sex, alcohol, reckless adventures, and more friends. Because more is better right!

Sometimes it's not just F.Y.I. It all landed me into worse off predicaments in the end. This only fueled more hatred in myself and for others who were living carefree without the internal pain that I was feeling. I call this the "Hamster Wheel Effect" when you keep doing the same things that keep you going nowhere fast, yet you feel if you stop that it all will come crashing down. You know the facade, persona, reputation well everything. In hindsight, I should have gotten off that damn wheel! Fortunately, I did eventually, but not before it would come at a great cost to me.

On a side note, the problem in our society is that there are not enough safe spaces to get this out. When you talk like this you are now labeled crazy, emotional, erratic or an outcast. Listen, if you or anybody you know is going through this downward spiral of negativity, please get yourself or them help. We are humans and we are not meant to do it alone. To continue where I left off, I did not see it coming because I did not seek help, my pride would not let me.

"Pride comes before the fall" is a very true saying and I got to experience it firsthand. In this state of mind, I became full of despair and hopelessness. Living another day became a burden, I sometimes wished I wouldn't wake up. I contemplated suicide and even attempted it. I was playing a dangerous game flirting with the idea of death. "We all are going to die anyway" or "We all got to go sometimes" became my thought process. I sucked at life for thinking this stupid shit looking back, but at the time it was a reality for me. This would become my new normal and what little did I know of the monsters I would face ahead.

CHECK THE MIRROR:

YOU ARE THE ENEMY

I AM THE MONSTER YOU CREATED...DEAL WITH IT!!!

I don't care and I don't give a fuck became the attitude. Sounds disrespectful and messed up right? I know because at times I messed over and disrespected myself as well as others. The world is a cruel place and the nice guy finishes last. The bad guys win and get what they want, I guess I've officially lived long enough to see myself become the villain. Hate it or love it but you created it, I thought. I started to embody the negativity as if it were my true make up, almost embracing it as if it were my nature. Well looking back, it is very much a part of me, but it is not the real me. Now what do I mean by the real me? The negative side of me stemmed from my ego failing me, but the real me is beyond such low levels of being. I started to take this trip down a rabbit whole I would soon come to regret.

The enemy I was looking for was with me the whole time taunting me, following me, sleeping with me and this sucker had the audacity to be living in me. Can you believe this entity, it doesn't even pay rent, well I guess when you voluntarily allow it in and make it comfortable it's considered squatter's rights huh? The dark became a comfortable place, wait that's a lie, it became a familiar place and I accepted it for what it was. I wanted to take the hurt I felt and let it out. I grew tired of holding it in.

Remember when I talked about the façade, well it came crumbling down when it was too much to contain within myself. I started to express my pain outwardly and the more I did it the more I became comfortable with it. Talk about building a new habit right. You know the thing you do until it's stuck on repeat. Yeah! That became the way I would express my negative perspective of the world. The real messed up part was I was justifying my newly adopted way of thinking by saying things like "I could always be worse" or "there are people worse than me". This gave me an outlet to live without a care of what I was doing to people. Deep down I wanted to be a better person, but let's face it being what I considered bad felt kind of good. It's the instant gratification we get from doing something on the edge that gives us the thrills. Since the rest of life sucked, I felt hey I might as well get my jollies off doing crazy, wild, and reckless things for personal gain. Like I said there were moments when this was beneficial and when this was not. Listen, let me tell you something. If something seems too good to be true, well dammit; guess what? It really is too good to be true.

It is a consequence to everything we do, good or bad. The consequence is usually determined by the state of the action you took, whether a positive action or a negative one. Lesson here people - take a lot of calculated positively charged actions in your life to receive positive consequences. Do not overdo the positive, because you still need to be aware of the negative as well, since both energies exist in this world. I played the blame game quite often for my actions, meaning I was not at a stage where I was quite ready to own up to them. But man did it feel good not to be responsible for them, well you know until you have to be. Here is the thing.

When you get away with something in one area of your life; you think it will not catch up to you. The funny thing is, in the other areas of your life where you are trying to be decent, is where your consequences will catch up to you. Welcome to the wonderful world of karma everyone and all of it joys. Well, karma is a bitch and this is avoidable. It is the explosion of your past actions coming back to bite you in the present time. If you think you can beat karma let me tell you that your chances are slim and even more so compounded the longer it is avoided. There is an exception to every rule and you better learn what those exceptions are because karma is an exceptional character. Not many can beat it at its own game. The best thing you can do is own up to your actions, make amends and move on. The question is what if you do not consider your actions to be negative but you are the creation and the creator? You created the monster in your mind and then acted in character playing out this monster. A creator would never make such a monster, oh yeah, well ask Dr. Frankenstein how he feels about that!

WAIT… I CREATED THE MONSTER INSIDE

No, I am not to blame for this, it is society, authorities, environment, media, and everyone else. The thing is these parts play a role, but we are the main character. We decide to commit to this role by making a choice. What needs to be corrected is our source of information in which we base our choices. If we knew the right information, we could make better choices. To obtain this information, we must seek it out, because some of us are not privileged enough to have this information at our fingertips. Also, accept that you are a creator whether a good or bad one that is up to you. We create using our mind and if we are not careful, we may produce creations that we deem undesirable. Now since we are not perfect, we will make mistakes but the thing we must do is learn from those mistakes, so we lessen the chances of making them again.

By the time I realized I was the monster I was already too far gone. My thought had become my belief and my belief had become my truth. When you make something your truth then you live by that truth, but is it true, if it is based on a lie? You know the lie that you told yourself. This is who I am now. This is just the way my life is. Nobody understands my life. I didn't choose this for myself. These statements are all victimizing phrases we tell ourselves to rationalize our negative thought process. If you are telling yourself these phrases, then you reinforce the truth you decided to tell yourself. I was telling myself these kinds of phrases and the more I did the more I held true to them. I created an unwanted reality where I attracted more negativity, more pain, more unwanted consequences, and I became the monster created by my own thoughts. I directly and indirectly hurt people by speaking carelessly, acting irrationally, behaving selfishly and willfully being ignorant. This was a spiritual crime against me that bled out into humanity. I had no idea what true spirituality was, but I would come to know it well. I will save those tales for later.

Back to the situation, at the current state I was in I had to do one thing and that was face the mirror. I was hiding because I was afraid of what I would find, and I had every right to be. See I was the devil in the flesh, maybe not the worst devil but the devil nonetheless. The thing we never consider is letting go, we tend to hold on until we can't any longer. That is when we look in the mirror and break it because we realize we hate what we have become.

FACING THE MIRROR: I DON'T LIKE WHAT I'VE BECOME

First off, let me start by saying I didn't break any mirrors! Replacing mirrors is expensive, and I did not have enough money to be that dramatic. Then again, I was dramatic at times, I would punch brick walls, car doors, property that was not mine and hit myself every now and then in the ribs or gut. I wanted to pinch myself to see if I were alive because I could not believe the condition, I was in was real. I would drink to escape, go out partying to feel free and use sexual promiscuity to assert dominance and chase pleasure. I was not addicted to anything but escaping my current hell. Living life became so dark and cold I would seek the light and warmth of others to feel alive only to pollute it with my negative vibes. I was allowing my darkness to absorb the light. I would get mad at myself for not being able to rectify my circumstances. This cycle of wanting better for myself but falling short because of self-imposed limitations became a roller coaster ride. I would never recommend anyone get on.

The truth in life is I was not doing the things I wanted to do, I was being somebody else for others. It was not true to me like I wanted to be. I was merely just fragmenting myself. I worked at jobs that paid me well enough to stay but I wanted to do more in my life. I wanted better health for myself but gave myself every reason to let my weight get out of control. I wanted better relationships but was so tired of putting my heart on the line that I became heartless. I wanted a meaning to my life but fell for the slavery of materialism and by the time I found out I entered slavery it was too late.

My ego told me the life I was living was cool. I mean I had money, clothes, cars, cell phones, jewelry, a condo, and popularity. The truth is I had money only on paper, the clothes were discounted, those cars were financed, the cell phones were leased, the jewelry was a waste, the condo was shared with a roommate and my popularity was based on bullshit. Now I had people who cared for me and loved me, but my ego could not see that.

THE EGO

"The Ego" was busy trying to be accepted and liked. After all, they say it's not what you know, it's who you know. Well if you have the wrong connections, guess what, you don't know the right people. It all boils down to I was living a lie and I wanted more but I was settling. I got comfortable and I justified my life by comparing myself to others. Like I am doing okay I got this and this, they don't have it. I worked to get this myself. Nobody helped me. I beat statistics. I'm supposed to be dead or in jail, so there is that. All that conditioned thinking was exactly what would lead to my internal demise. I damn near destroyed my external world too. If I could tell you one thing it is to never turn your back on the real you for no one, not your parents, friends, significant other, strangers, organizations, or your ego. Your ego really is not a bad thing; it is what you fill your ego with that makes it bad. If I had a do over, I certainly would use my ego accordingly.

"The Ego" should never be let off the leash; it should be under control the entire time. You will need it in your life, but it should never run your life. The Ego can't die, it's a part of you. You must learn to subdue the Ego. If precautions aren't taken then, there will come a day where you will hate yourself. I guarantee it! The mirror shows all and if you don't check it often enough you may look up to find a distorted self-image. I hated the part I was playing but I accepted it and that was the biggest mistake.

Do yourself a favor - never take what life throws at you lying down. Fight for it! Keep your guard up! Stick and move (that's boxing terminology)! If you lose, you will live to fight another day, but you stand no chance in winning by cowering away in the corner or lying face down. That is when another decision must be made. Say to yourself: I am tired of waiting to be saved; I am going to save myself; I am going to face my fears; I will overcome them! If only it were that simple. How are you going to save yourself, if you do not know who you are anymore, or better yet, you never knew? Wish I could tell you it gets easier from here; but it does not. Saving yourself will be one of the hardest things you ever do, but the amount of strength and wisdom you gain is immeasurable. So how did I save myself you ask? Well turn the page if you dare to take this journey of trial and tribulation with me.

SAVE YOURSELF FROM THE

HELL YOU CREATED

NO ONE IS COMING TO SAVE YOU

Realize this, no one is going to swoop down out of the sky to come and rescue you. Although when you read it in the comics it sounds good. You are going to have to learn to be your own hero starting from the ground floor. But I don't have superpowers. Yeah, I know but you will learn your powers in time but right now you need a plan! Have you ever asked yourself why you were not taught to be your own savior, champion, or hero? I often asked myself why I wasn't taught this! If I would have known to not be solely dependent on things outside of myself, I could have done something about my circumstances sooner. This is why I felt compelled to write this book in order to help others learn how to save themselves.

Often, we suffer not just from lack of knowledge but from not knowing it sooner. Imagine if you knew who you were sooner what could you accomplish. Instead, we know about everything but self and that is exactly why we have become victims of our own circumstances. We need to dive deep into our psyche to find that super powered person we can become to free ourselves from the hell around us. Even more, free ourselves from the hell inside of us. Pull your head out of the clouds! Stop looking at organizations and people around and start looking within. It is there where your starting point should be, you must put in the "self-work" before you go outside of yourself for more answers. Okay so how does this all come together you may be wondering. Well, let's take a look at some steps we need to identify so we know what to do when this darkness arises (i.e. "The Hell Creation").

FIRST KNOW THE HELL YOU LIVE IN ORDER TO ESCAPE IT

You must know your hell, in order to escape. People often say, 'how did I get here' or 'why does this keep happening to me'? You'd know 'the how' if you searched within. It's because this is the hell you were busy creating in your mind little by little. The 'Hell creation' is part thoughts, part beliefs, part egotism, part energy, part feelings and part actions. Alright so, the 'Hell creation' at the ground floor is your thoughts, where you begin to wonder what could be the worst thing that could happen to you. Examples are: 'what if I am forever hated', 'what if I lose all my money, lose my job, lose my business', 'what if I lose my loved one(s),' or 'what if my reputation is ruined?'. Get the picture now. Thinking these things aren't necessarily bad as it could empower you to learn to be more likable, watch your money better, spend time with loved ones, protect your reputation, etc.

Now what happens when you move to level 1 which is your beliefs. It is here in our beliefs that further our thoughts on certain topics or not. What I am saying is if we put belief behind the thoughts we had about a certain thing, then those thoughts may start to get entertained quite often in our minds. Now this belief is starting a thought process which dives deeper into the thought itself. If you become used to this thought process, you will create a habit of thinking about this thought often.

Next is level 2, in this level "the Ego" decides if this believed thought is a threat or not. If it is determined to not be a threat the Ego will let it go but if it is determined to be a threat the Ego will go code red and start to devote energy to stopping the threat. The Ego does not want to be killed and if it feels threatened it will go ape shit to stop anything from happening to it. By the way your true self is just observing the thoughts while your ego, which is usually louder, is saying hey it's either kill or be killed!

Then there is level 3 called energy, where this power is distributed either toward light force or dark force. Now, if you are having dark thoughts, this energy is more prone to going toward dark forces within and around you. You may start to view and criticize yourself and others in a negatively harsh way. By transferring power to this force, it can start to suck you further into it which leads to the next level.

Feelings are level 4 and on this lovely level is where you feel emotions. This level involves sensitivity that can impact your world in the mental and the physical sense. See, feelings can either enable or disable you from doing anything. If you are headed on the path to darkness more than likely this will enable fears and a scarcity mindset mentally. Physically this will disable you from conquering your fears through actions, also it can cause stress, bodily pains, fatigue, tiredness, slower movement, down states etc.

Finally, there is level 5 which is actions. When in action, we move in the physical world either in a positive or negative direction. These directions are based on perception. For instance, a person scared of heights may perceive going on a roller coaster as a negative thing while a thrill seeker may perceive it as a positive thing in their book. If we are negatively charged, there is likely a chance that we will take little to no action in the physical world. Now there are times where we need to slow down or rest but too much of this would be considered a negative action. However, if we are in a constant negative orientation, then nothing would ever get done due to no action ever being taken. There are levels to this but know how to maneuver on these levels, otherwise you will find yourself falling to the ground floor again. The saying goes, "dust yourself off and try again", but then again you don't really want to keep making the same mistakes and repeating the same cycles now do you? The lessons to be learned are: to observe your thoughts; practice your beliefs; shut down your ego; and unlock your true self. Also, give energy to what you can control, express your feelings - just don't stay in them, and take relentless action to strive toward your purpose and goals.

IT'S ALL OR NOTHING: DO SOMETHING, ANYTHING TO SAVE YOURSELF

You do not need a superpower to have a plan. Now that you know the levels to the layout of your Hell, it is time to create that plan. Prepare for the plan and do whatever you can to not go further in the dark space. Simply put - run!!!!! Okay, you probably are looking for a specific step by step break down to a plan. Let me ask you. Do you think life will happen in very specific steps? No, life just happens and I would suggest reversing everything you were doing. That is right! I said it! Instead of doing your normal routine that empowers these negative behaviors, you must break the behavioral cycle by being courageous enough to do something different. For instance:

- If you feel pissed off, don't go drink alcohol. Instead go lift weights or even better hit a punching bag until your heart's content.

- If you feel alone, do not stay alone thinking about it. Go see a loved one or friend that really makes you feel good. If they aren't available, call and if that doesn't work then go to a place where like-minded people are who are interested in similar things as you. When your thoughts start to bring you down, watch or read material that will help to combat the mental funk. If thoughts are running through your head, write them down and once written close the journal or crumble the page and throw it away.

- If your beliefs are clouded by your ego, take a hard look in the mirror and ask yourself these questions. Are my beliefs based on other people's opinions? Does this belief serve me or does it move me? Will this belief move me forward or set me back? Why do I believe this belief about myself? Did someone give me this belief or did I give myself this belief?

- If your energy is up do not go to the club where validation is the currency to feel valued. Instead read that book you always wanted to read or start that project you were interested in.

- If your energy is low, do not attempt to force yourself to do anything. Take a nap, meditate or decompress by getting a massage. The key here is to do something different. Doing the same things will get you the same results.

- If you are an extrovert, try being an introvert or vice versa.

- If you like going out to hear a band, try staying in and learning how to play an instrument.

- If you like traveling to other countries try traveling to other parts of your own city, surely there is still more to explore there.

- If you get enjoyment from eating out, try cooking for a change. You may learn that you are pretty good at it.

Again, I repeat, do not get into a habit of doing the same things over and over because it will get you nowhere and even worse; if you do nothing, it will leave you in the same place. You might say, "But why should I give up what instantly makes me feel good and makes me happy?" Then don't take my advice and do what you want. Just know you aren't ready to be saved because you enjoy pretending you are fine. Remember that is a choice. We are here to grow and expand, so being the same only feels good for a while until life forces growth out of us.

You can either go with the current of life or get dragged by it. What option do you choose? Oh, I have your attention again I see. Well, I am glad you are choosing the path of least resistance. Trust me, the path of pretenders sucks big time; take my word for it. I tried that and wasted time, money, energy and effort. Repeating the same cycles and absolutely going nowhere isn't living life - it is just existing in it. I'm still haunted by the demons from my past. If I would have done something different sooner, then I could have gone with the tide but instead I went against it and eventually I was swallowed by it. Don't think of yourself as special because nature always wins. My natural ass got handed to me on more than one occasion in life. If you want to be saved, ask yourself what would a real-life hero do and go look up people who embody those qualities. That is a good starting place on top of the other suggestions mentioned.

There is plenty of material on real life heroes from documentaries to autobiographies. Hey! If you can access one in person even better, go to see them. Choose anyone you look up to, even mature family and friends and ask them how they would get through this trying time. Never be afraid to ask for help. That was a huge mistake of mine that would eventually cost me everything. I still sleep with my demons but I never give them a warm bed because I hog all the covers now! It wasn't always like that, sometimes they would kick me out of my own bed, literally I fell out of the bed from nightmares of my life falling apart. Tell me, do you sleep with your demons?

SLEEPING WITH YOUR

DEMONS

THOUGHTS KEEP RUNNING THE MIND

The mind is a terrible thing to waste. Who here has heard that before? While that is true, sometimes you may want to take your brain out of your head and put it in the trash. When the thoughts keep running in your mind and you can't seem to hit the off switch, it makes you wish you could just get rid of it all together. A mind that cannot have quiet time can have no peace and a mind without peace is doomed for insanity. The off switch has to be pulled immediately so that the mind can reset. It is not as simple as it sounds.

In order to switch your mind off, you must be okay with surrendering your thoughts and letting go. How do you do that? Well, that differs for everyone. It is not a one size fits all answer. A good start is shutting down thoughts out of your head. If you never shut them out, you will never have a peaceful rest when you sleep at night. Those demons get louder in the dark and they like to keep you up. Besides, they feed off of your torment. Tools that can help are writing, recording, or talking your thoughts out. None of these tools will cure this condition overnight, however things will gradually get a little more tolerable and eventually better. Trust me if thoughts are let out, they can be freed and you won't have to feel that heavy weight on your shoulders. If you like to hold on to misery then that is addiction at its finest my friend and the substance being abused is toxic thoughts.

Pick whichever tool is more convenient for you, but I also encourage you to use every tool at your disposal. The more you use these tools the more release mechanisms you'll have to get the toxic thoughts out of your head. Other release tools are meditation, boxing, running, weight-lifting, screaming (war cry), music, dancing or being outdoors in nature. These are just a few to name, as stated before it will be different for everyone because we all will want to release differently. I strongly encourage releasing in a healthy way. For example, using sex to release by sleeping with someone you have no attachments to or feelings for. There is a possibility this may have negative consequences, as a result of the interaction, which can lead to increased stress levels and give those demons more to feed off of. Another example is using gambling, as a way to escape negative thinking: "If I feel like a winner, I can change my circumstances! I just have to play big to win big!" All of a sudden, you are in the hole and in even more debt than when you started. Here, again, this is just compounding the stress.

Never put yourself in a position where the risk outweighs the reward, especially being in this negative state of being. Pick safe bets and use tools that will lessen or completely remove the chances of compounding your stress levels. Hopefully, these tips can help you get on the right track and slow thoughts down from running to a walking pace.

THE NIGHTMARES

Here I want to address the nightmares specifically. They will drive anyone crazy seeing that it's a reminder that you are not in a peaceful state. Nightmares can be read many ways but they are happening for a reason. Here is a list of some of those different ways. Nightmares can mean you have not dealt with something and you are running from it. Also, they can mean you have a great fear, guilt or sense of regret. It may also mean you have not learned a lesson so it keeps showing the same thing over and over until something clicks. Then they can be visuals showing your perception of the world and how grim you believe it to be. These are just a few ways in which nightmares surface, but one of my favorites is the nightmare where you have no choice but to stand up for yourself and fight. In this one, it may be a reoccurring dream, but once the foe being faced is beaten, you wake up with a sense of relief feeling courageous and confident. Nightmares do not have to be all bad. The key is to figure them out and what they mean. To lessen the chances of nightmares, we must do things while awake that will bring peace while sleeping. Activities that garner confidence, trust in self, bravery, awareness, possibility, openness, and self-actualization will allow feelings of empowerment to come about. What to do here is place yourself in uncomfortable and new situations that will bring out these qualities inside of you. You will fail but failure is good. Just keep going and once you finally overcome the challenging activity, the achievement will be well worth it. Now, what will this do for those nightmares? Well, put it this way; what can be done while awake can be done in dreamland or vice versa. Those nightmares are just lessons that must be studied so that the test can be passed. If you do nothing to stop these nightmares, they will grow darker and feed the demons more. This, in turn, will reward no peace - just even more torment and misery.

The nightmares will then manifest into the outer world and become real for the ego. When "the Ego" feels threatened, we already know it will do whatever it can to protect itself as we learned earlier. It will even shut off your ability to adapt and overcome because it will be focusing your attention on the problem and not the solution. Nightmares and "the Ego" must be subdued, otherwise, they will wreak havoc in our lives causing drama and chaos to ensue.

DEMONS NEVER SLEEP SO SLEEP WITH THEM

Alright, so you still can't sleep huh? Well let me tell you something, learn to sleep with your demons. You can't sleep because you have not made peace with your demons. They are there as warnings and reminders of what you should not do. At first it will feel like they are haunting you and to some degree they are, how else are they going to scare you back on the right track. If you never face anything, how will you know what is morally right or wrong or how will you know what is right or wrong for you? The demons are given power by your fears.

Once you acknowledge what you fear, you can then begin the process of overcoming. Further along in the overcoming process demons will grow weaker until the point where you can sleep with them like teddy bears. If you are like me, you will kick them out of the bed from time to time to remind them who's in charge. The demons never really sleep. They are either in dreams while sleeping or in daydreams while awake. Heck, even some people or places in life will remind you of the demons. What you want to do is stop running from them and get to know them. This will be the only way to move forward. To take down the demons you must acknowledge, accept, take action, commit and reflect often.

Acknowledge their presence and do not pretend they don't exist in your life. If you have a problem, do you act like it doesn't exist or do you pay attention to it. By paying attention you can set an intention to fix the problem. Listen, if you do not give them the attention, they deserve they will just continue to keep ruining your life until you do. Leave it up to "The Ego" and you will be tormented forever simply because the ego is self-absorbed. Ego does not want to feel as if it is incapable or weak. It will simply ignore issues until it can't anymore and by then it is too late.

Next, accept the fact that they are there, you are the reason why and that this is a problem that needs to be addressed. Acceptance is hard, but so is life, people who accept take ownership and responsibility. Once acceptance occurs, the feeling of relief becomes present. You no longer carry the weight of unacceptance and can finally ask the question what do I do now? In the next phase, 'taking action' is where you dig in. Start looking for different methods that suit you, talk to people who face similar challenges, find content on your current issue, do plenty of self-talk or record your thoughts. Take whatever action needed until you find your outlet and stick with that until you feel the need to change your approach. Once you have found that outlet and settled on an approach, commit to it.

Committing requires diligent focus on the matter and never taking your finger off the pulse of what you committed to. The minute you let up, it is like the flood gates open and the problem starts to grow again feeding the demons and so on. Committing requires attention and a keen eye, never take your eye off the prize. What is the prize you ask - your sanity! Finally reflect often. This one is to me the most important. If there is no reflection, there is no direction. If you choose not to look back on mistakes you've made and things you've done, you cannot possibly know how to move forward. Without reflection, we go in circles.

We have plenty of negative reoccurrences and we dig ourselves deeper each time. Once the hole is deep enough and you see no light, the darkness will take hold again. It becomes so familiar being there that you may find yourself taking up permanent residency. I am sure you do not want to go down this road. Not many make it back.

DEMONS AREN'T SO SCARY ONCE YOU FACE THEM

You have learned a lot about demons so now what are you going to do about your own? They don't just go away! You have to work on them like it's a job. An Exorcist would say I will exorcise your demons. I say exercise your own demons. Make them work for you! As far as I know, they pay no rent, they pay no bills and they are annoying. If this is the case then make them work to be in your presence, let them teach you some things and show you the problem areas in your mentality. They are not so scary, if you become heavily acquainted with them. Most times they are just looking for some attention and in the long run paying attention to them works in your favor. They will show you the error of your ways and teach you (sometimes the hard way) how to correct them. They aren't the boogie man - you are!

If you do not gain control of yourself and your thoughts, then you become a monster. We already know what that can lead to. Being in fear of the demons will not change your circumstances but facing them head-on eventually will. Never turn your back to the demons, never give them a chance to catch you off guard. Face them! Take a stance and acknowledge their presence so they know you have no intentions of backing down.

SLAYING DRAGONS

AND

SOMETIMES HYDRAS

HIDING IN THE CLOSET OF YOUR MIND

"This is not real! You're not real! This isn't happening to me!" are the thoughts going through your head. The enemy that you see is very real, but to you only. Pretending your situation is not real won't help. It will only add to the troubles that are already there. You can hide in the recesses of your mind, but you will have to come out sometimes. That problem that you are putting off is like a virus. If you don't take care of it soon, it will keep spreading until it out numbers your defenses. I wish I would have known what I'm about to say sooner, "If under attack, when given the opportunity, kill the enemy in its tracks." To retreat means stepping back to regroup and creating a strategy to seek higher grounds.

On the other hand, hiding means holding position and seeking no interaction with the opposer until the battle is over. If hiding is your battle strategy, that will only give the enemy more time to close in, covering every position and taunting you while doing so until captured. When a dragon of a thought arises to set you ablaze, take cover, if need be, but find the means to slay it! Kill it without fail, as soon as possible or it will come back fiercer than ever to take you out. These negative thoughts I call "dragons" because they have a tendency to come out of nowhere and wreak havoc almost immediately. They catch your mind off guard and will have the mind racing and running scared. Nine times out of ten, you weren't prepared for your 'first dragon' thought because it was a new experience. Well guess what, you better go to 'dragon slayer' academy real quick to get prepared for the next onslaught. These thoughts grow strong, if they aren't put down right away. The only way to stop it is through preparation. Know your enemy well. Don't run from it and besides, no one can run forever.

CAN'T RUN FOREVER

If running is the strategy to fend the dragons off, then I'd hate for one to encounter a hydra when they come out to play. In Greek mythology, 'hydra' is a fictitious poisonous monster with multiple heads that grow back when you cut them off. Oh, and they don't play fair! I call recurring negative thoughts ``hydras" because it seems like there is no end to these thoughts. When you finally get a chance to catch your breath from fending one off, another one comes back again and again. These suckers are trouble with a capital T. They will make daily life hard if their weakness is not found. How can their weakness be found if you are in hiding? See now why running isn't a good idea. Facing it is the only option.

Unlike the dragons that can be killed relatively easily, hydras tend to regenerate quickly and come back with double the ferocity. The only way of getting rid of them is to stop their source of regeneration or obliterate them entirely. Running is temporary because no matter where you go, they will find you. Running is a tactic to lure it, distract it or take temporary cover from it. But never make running a strategy.

Now, to take this away from fantasy land and put this in non-fiction terminology. We have thousands of thoughts per day some are minuscule, grand, important, unimportant, high priority, low priority, good or bad, relevant, irrelevant, smart or stupid, desired or undesired and so on. Get the picture? With all of that going on in the head, the ones that have the most impact are your emotional thoughts. Any thought we think of and tie emotion to, tends to hold in our mind. The real question to ask here is are our emotions in check? If not, then they can lead to self-destructive thoughts and the worst is having them reoccur.

PAST PAINS AFFECT PRESENT SANITY

The most important time is "NOW" but the majority of us live in the past. We wonder why our present is in shambles, not realizing it is because we haven't let certain things in our past go. I know all too well how the past can be haunting. The only solution here is to go back and I mean way back to the very beginning. Go as far as you can recall and start from there. You have to identify the origins of the enemy within. We all have origin stories within our inner selves. The inner-self is based out of thought, experience, and imagination. Remember when you were a little child? Think back - recall anything? Maybe as a little boy you wanted to be a superhero or as a little girl you wanted to be a princess.

You make up a story of how you want things to go using power of thought. You imagine how the role is being played out in life and then you live the experience through fantasy. You may even do this to a point where it all starts to feel like reality. This is an origin story. Now let's say something tragic or traumatic happens in your life. It then becomes hard to shake those thoughts centered around that event. What happens next is that you begin to imagine it from different vantage points and relive the experience over and over again. It may sound crazy, but this happens when we do not have a defense mechanism in place to properly deal with these traumatizing emotional events and originating thoughts. With no sound defense, it becomes hard to play offense.

In order to build a defense, you must learn who you're defending against. Tracing things back to those very first thoughts centered around a particular event is crucial. Ask yourself questions like, "Was it as bad as I'm making it seem? Can someone else have it worse than me?

Was I a part of the problem? If so, what role did I play? Was I aware or unaware? Was I naïve or did I know the risk? What could I have done?" This questioning process sucks because it almost seems as if the problem falls on you. Trust me, what this questioning process allows you to do is put things into perspective. Once things are in perspective they can then be dealt with accordingly. Understanding the part you played in it, is crucial because it helps with acknowledging what happened and makes you aware. When you are aware then it's less likely you will be in a situation like that again because you will have learned recognition.

Recognition helps to recall previous encounters with people or things. It is important we use recognition because it can get us out of unwanted spaces. Like the saying goes "you better recognize". This is the only way to prevent a recurrence is to recognize what is going on around you and within you. I recall times of being bullied when I was younger both verbally and physically. At first, it would terrify me to see the bully and I tried to stay away from them as much as I could. I thought, 'I am nice. Why do they pick on me or what did I do to them?' I really started to believe that I was the problem. I said things like: 'It's because I'm fat. Skinny people don't have this problem. If I were skinny, I wouldn't have to deal with this.' I started to submit myself to the bullying because a part of me felt I deserved it. I would cry, get angry and get whooped. I had conformed to this is just the way it was.

Until one day I made up my mind, I am sick of this shit! I knew when I was going to get bullied, I knew the place and I had a plan. One time I recall vividly is the infamous "bathroom bullies" incident. These two knuckleheads would beat me up damn near every day for a while and I took it. Then one day I knew, when the teacher had us line up to go into the washroom two at a time, it was on. The rules were to line up along the bathroom wall in pairs. Two would go in, if one was done early then he'd come out and the teacher would send only one in so that it was always two people in at one time. If we had to hurry up so we could get to the next period, the teacher sent in 2 instead of one. Well, just my luck that when my partner went out one of the bullies would come in. When I came out of the stall, the other one was coming through the door. They laughed and teased me as I was washing my hands. I dried my hands and started to walk out as the big one said where are you going? Before I knew it the small one grabbed me while the big one punched me. Since I was a chubby kid, I was able to use my weight to throw the little one off and kick the big one dead in the nuts. Yes, his jingle bells! He screamed and hollered while I laughed and smiled. For the first time, I stood up for myself and it felt pretty damn good.

Now I am not condoning violence but at a certain point you have to say enough is enough. If you don't stand up for yourself, who else will? I just wanted peace. I just wanted my dignity, and I was tired of being the victim. Because I was at a Christian school, we both got a whooping from the principal. The only difference was, he was crying from two pains, the one from down below and the one from the belt coming across his behind. I gladly took my whooping with the belt because I finally didn't feel like a loser. After that we all sat and watched a movie in the cafeteria/auditorium and the teacher made him say sorry. From that point on we became cool.

The point of this story is to let you know that I became aware and started to recognize what was going on around me and within me. I knew how I felt and I was tired of the same thing happening to me especially because I had done nothing wrong. I knew the time and place where situations were likely to happen and all I had to do was decide what I was going to do about it. I knew the opponent I was defending against and I knew how the opponent made me feel. I had gained perspective over the situation and from there I was able to handle it accordingly. I no longer chose to live in the past. This is just the way it is and that I deserve this as a fat kid. I decided in the present moment to act differently which rewarded me a different outcome than the previous ones I was used to. I decided to defend myself, I decided to fight!

FIGHTING IS THE ONLY OPTION LEFT

Listen, these dragons and hydras are coming one day and making sure you prepare as much as possible should be a singular focus. Truth is nothing can prepare you one hundred percent for the battles ahead. Here is the thing, would you rather know something useful, have some tools, some sort of skills, some awareness and preparation than nothing at all? Sure, you would, so don't fool yourself. When should you start training? RIGHT NOW!

At this exact moment, take some time to think over what you have read up until this point and start devising a strategy for your life. Use some of the things you have learned from the previous chapters to start putting the playbook together. This can wait no longer! You don't deserve this! It's up to you to believe you deserve better, not anyone else! People will help you fight, but only if they see you fighting for your life. No one is coming just to pick you up and dust you off. This is a job for you. It's your life - your mission.

Plan ahead! Trust your instincts! Follow your gut! Take action! Participate in your own life! I can't make any guarantees besides this - if you do nothing, you will keep getting what you are getting, which is nothing at all. Fighting just to be fighting is pointless but fighting for a just cause is everything. Your life should be as just of a cause as any. You must arm yourself with your values, morals, and principles. You must train the mind for clarity and focus. Train the body to take the necessary action. Train your emotions so they won't get the best of you and express them in healthy outlets. Train your spirit so that it won't die out and fade away on you. Above all else, practice getting to know yourself while training so you will know what you are fighting for. Whom you are fighting for is your inner self. This is crucial because you do not want to be an empty shell of a person. Do not put off training, for if you do, great suffering will come upon you that could have been avoided. At birth you fought to get here - now in life you fight to be here. ARM YOURSELF!

EVERYDAY IS A BATTLE...WAR IS FAR FROM OVER

Ladies and gentlemen, I wish that I could tell you that yes it will all be fine after this current battle in your life, but I would be lying. See, the fight is an ongoing occurrence because as long as you live you will always have to face yourself (i.e., choices you have made, decisions you regret, consequences that were sown and past traumas that resurface are all things that will come back to challenge you).

The more reflecting you do - the more prepared you will be for when the inner battle returns. The road ahead is long, sometimes lonely and being a traveler can be tiresome. But would you rather be tired walking the path or stagnant and completely lost? No war was ever won without sacrifice, perseverance, heart, determination, and conviction of one's belief. We all should take time to remember the past battles and wars to prepare us for the ones yet to come. "Life is the ultimate struggle, but it's worth every step in the journey of discovery."

HERO'S JOURNEY...WAIT I'M

NOT HEROIC

HEROICS NOT FOR ME

We often assume that to be a hero we need some kind of special uniform, symbol and a superpower. When we look at heroism this way, we say, 'you know what, I am going to leave it up to one of those other guys.' That is understandable but what happens when you need saving? Are you just going to leave it up to the other guys? That just made you think, didn't it? Don't worry. That made me think too. We often put the heroics in other people's hands because we don't want to do the dirty work in our own lives. Plus, we can just blame them for not doing a good enough job.

Listen up, we can no longer just put off our problems on other people and blame them if we refuse to fully participate in our own life. Let me tell you something, it may be easier to put things off on others but in the long run you lose. The reason you lose is because it takes away your ability to solve your own problems and ultimately weakens you. Partnering with others on your problem is a better way. Think of it as being a sidekick if you will. Sidekicks watch the back of those helping them to become better heroes. See where I am going with this? Seeking out mentorship, help or guidance is better than just passing the ball and hoping the star will score every time. Play your part because heroes get tired too.

Playing your role does not require anything special except it does require participation. What can you do to help your situation that is well within your control? For example, you may consistently be the top producer driving revenue for the company you work at until one day the company decides to take a completely different route and replaces the old product for a new one you have no clue about. Now your production goes down and so does your revenue. Who is to blame here? It's the company because they changed without warning and there should have been better implementation! I get it, but did you ever ask why the company did that? Did you reach out to anyone for assistance? Did you search for training that could improve your knowledge of this new product? If not, there was a lack of heroics on your part. You could have saved your own day or at least participated. Sometimes our egos can get in the way that we believe it should always be us at the top because we earned it. But hey things change, companies change, people change, life will change and so should you. Inspire others to do the same through your actions because they may one day look to you for guidance.

A HERO IS A CHARACTER SO WHO'S YOURS

It is often said that most times heroes display strong character. So, what is a character? Well, in comic books it is the fiction-based person drawn up from a script. In reality, traits make up a person's character. That could sound confusing so let's dive into it. If strong character is what you are after, then building a strong inner foundation is key. Most heroes are not pushovers. Even the weakest among them will fight back if their back is against the wall.

Character is how the person carries themselves through life. Some people have a victimizing way of going through life. For others, they may be stubborn and aggressive. For heroes, it is often they are courageous, confident, caring, and selfless. These tend to be desirable character traits when it comes to saving people and yes even saving themselves. Your character in life is the best thing you can offer someone else. This is not the perfect gift, but it is the most vulnerable and truthful part of us. If we practice building strong character within ourselves, we can then give in a powerful way to others. Some heroes give us hope, inspiration, high energy, thoughtfulness, kindness and show us how to strive for better. By you and me building better character we are then able to accomplish some impossible tasks both individually and collectively.

If you take the best parts of yourself and multiply that times ten what then would you look like? How would you talk, walk, work, love and live? I am just saying a hero is in all of us but first we must learn to be heroic. Even in the origin stories the heroes don't start out day one saving the day, it's a learning process. To begin saving yourself, you must be willing to go through the process of building a strong character. That requires you being brave enough to go into the unknown world of self-discovery.

NOBODY WANTS TO TAKE ADVICE FROM THE INEXPERIENCED

Do you want just anybody to help you? Not even you want advice from someone who is inexperienced in life. Once the process of building strong character has started, it is time to put in the work. Finding help and mentorship is a good start - someone who has already walked in the path you desire to be in. During this time, you are to take a back seat and learn. This is not your time to shine. You will have your moment - don't worry. We all want 'that moment' but 'that moment' comes at a cost.

The fee is discipline and sacrifice. Discipline and sacrifice are two valuable practices most underestimated actions we could ever exercise. But now I will add some new ingredients to the recipe which are faith, will and focus. Discipline, sacrifice, faith, will and focus will get you through anything. You are going to go 'through hell' or as we call it 'the dark space', to be a hero. You need to discipline yourself constantly to stay the course, move forward and to never waiver. You must sacrifice your time, efforts, leisure, comfort and pleasure to grow beyond where you currently are. You will need faith to see what is possible but not currently here in front of you. There needs to be a faith so strong in you that, even when others can't see the big picture, you feel like you are already there. Faith is belief beyond the physical plane of existence. You must have the will to push through the pain, the hardships and the trials that await you around every corner. Without a will of our own, we fall prey to someone else's.

Lastly, focus is needed to see only the path laid out in front of you and the destination that awaits. These five things (discipline, sacrifice, faith, will and focus) from this day need to become principles ingrained in your mind to be utilized in trying times and throughout your life, period. The level of achievement you will reach will be beyond your wildest dreams!

THE TRIUMPHANT RETURN

Waiting on that day when the sun will shine its brightest for you will seem like all your work was not done in vain. Your speech, your smile, your walk, your look, and your overall character will be different. That day will be where you know your worth and others know it too. Yes, that day will be a day of triumph. That moment is the moment you understand that life is bigger than you and that you, just as well as anyone else, deserve a shot at it. You return from the darkness and walk in your light of truth.

You have come here to this world to tell your story and stake your claim. Prior to this, your journey will have been all internal, but now your external journey really begins. You will begin to express who you really are outwardly without shame and be able to stand for yourself. This is because you have gone through and overcome all the trials inside of you that have held you back. When you return, it will be to enact something greater and to add value. This is where you emerge as a symbol, a role model, and a hero. You see you may not have the superpowers but what you will have is a strong sense of self and nobody can take that away from you. That strength will give you confidence to be unapologetically you but will give others the confidence in your abilities. When you return your mission becomes teaching others how to come out from the darkness and into the light of truth...their truth.

FLIP THE SCRIPT ON

NEGATIVE ENERGY

TURNING THE TABLES

You may have returned triumphantly but that does not mean there will not be battles ahead in your life. The demons we spoke of earlier will try to claw their way back into your life if you are not aware of them. They lurk in the dark recesses of your mind waiting for your moment of vulnerability so they can pull you back in. Do not ever get too high upon your horse that you believe you can never fall again. There is an old saying but it still holds true to this day: "When those times come when darkness starts to bloom again, you must be prepared mentally to turn the tables. In those moments you must be prepared with what I call 'triggers'".

These are powerful statements that acknowledge what is happening inside you. This allows you to face those 'boogie man' thoughts right then and there before they get out of hand. A trigger word, phrase or action are commands that prompt you to extinguish those negative thoughts. It is not like an affirmation which affirms who you are. Do not get the two mistaken. These words and actions should be said or made with conviction.

Once a thought comes up, you may say aloud or in your mind the words ``not today" with ferocity. Shaking your head, no, may also be another trigger that prompts the expelling of negative thoughts. If you find that you are vulnerable because of a current situation, it is usually best to observe your thoughts in the moment to search for the demonic thoughts before they sneak up on you. But hey, if you are caught off guard, you always have your triggers. Remember to not let negative thoughts last longer because they can blow up on you quickly and that is when you have to use another method in your arsenal called 'Channeling the Negativity'.

CHANNELING THE NEGATIVITY

When negative thoughts become big enough to run a 'muck' in your mind it is time to drain them of energy. When you channel, you must concentrate hard on what is happening within and use it physically on the outside. For example, if you are having a bad day and the events that occur lead you to thoughts about an ex, loss of a loved one, a time where you lost your job or anything that leads to painful experiences, maybe a trip to the gym may help. The gym is a great place to physically act out what you are feeling, and it is usually best to do your heaviest lifts these days. This will get all that negative energy out of you and release you from its grasps. Maybe you are an artist, then painting may be another way to get it out.

By aggressively marking up the canvas with each stroke of paint flying, you will feel yourself slowly start to let go. The point is to concentrate on that thought and use it to act out physically in a healthy way – thus releasing stress and anxiety. Know how not to use negativity to harm people! They didn't do anything to you! It was your thoughts getting the best of you. Remember, only you have the power to control your thoughts so why not do it the best way you know how.

'Channeling the negativity' is a tool for absorbing and releasing. Never, under any circumstances, should you hold on to that which does not serve you the best. 'Channeling the negativity' allows you to release positive thoughts in an expressive way. The actions you take while 'channeling' can sometimes turn into the most productive or creative moments in your life if done properly. Just remember that before you go start trying to break stuff or hurt someone, use this method to make advances in your life. If the thoughts have already started and have grown to take up massive space in your brain then there is only one thing left to do. Be still.

PRACTICING STILLNESS, DEEP OBSERVATION AND BREATHING

Alright so now you are up shit creek without a paddle, another old saying that still has relevance. When negative thoughts are not channeled in a proper way, they tend to expand and grow. Once they expand, you cannot run from them. Here are some suggestions on how to channel negative thoughts:

1. Find yourself a quiet place to think things through very deeply.

2. Observe each thought down to the details to make sense of what you are feeling.

3. Keep a journal or a voice recorder close by, if things get really intense. This way you can get them out of your head and record them. Making a record of thought requires you to capture these details and have a point of reference to refer to.

4. Close your eyes.

5. Breathe deeply. Deep breathing quiets the heart and causes you to focus, so much so that it takes attention away from the thoughts and puts it on just being. Deep breathing will calm the body so that there can be total concentration of the mind. The deeper your breathing is during stillness, the deeper you can go into observation of thoughts. This may take minutes to hours, but the point is to wage war on the mind and submerge yourself in thought.

6. The best defense is offense. In this case, do not emerge until you have made some sense of the negativity you feel. In doing this it stops the negative expansion and gives way to minimizing these thoughts.

7. Take time to celebrate the small wins. Reflect on what you did successfully so that you can repeat that success in the future.

8. Finally, be still! Do not carry on your day or week without practicing stillness, otherwise you may find yourself slowly slipping back into the darkness from which you came. The difference then was you fell because you were not armed with the right tools to protect yourself, but you are now. At this point you either use those tools or go back to being consumed by negativity again. My point is making time to settle the matter before it settles you!

YOU HAVE ARRIVED... PSYCH

IT'S NOT THAT EASY

Yay! You did it! That was only one battle and you learned how to flip the script but now guess what? More nonsense is on its way! Just because we make great strides does not mean the war is over. In fact, it is far from over. As long as there is life in you, you'll have to fight but the point is to find peace in the midst of the chaos. We often want to find the shortcut solution to our problem and hey if you just so happen to luck up, then good for you. But for the majority of us no such luck exists, it is either we learn to fall in love with suffering or make our beds and lay in them.

I would love to tell you that you made it and it is legit, but it is more like you made it through a round in a tournament. The question you may be thinking now is what do I do? Everything you have learned, up until this point, you simply rinse and repeat. There are plenty of other monsters in your closet that need to be addressed and the good news is that you already had some practice with some previously.

Instead of focusing on the victory, it is time to take your focus within. The real battles are the ones you are having inside of yourself and that will require you to take many trips within to see what new battle awaits. This process is called Self-Work which means to go inside of yourself to get rid of the thoughts, programs, behaviors, habits and beliefs that aren't serving you. It requires repetition to keep your demons in check.

Please do not make the mistake of believing that it's over. Staying sharp keeps you on your toes and ready for when that day arises when a negative thought enters your mind in which you can't afford to entertain. It is through lack of awareness that we least expect things to occur.

If we give up fighting for what we have built, it means it wasn't strong enough to stand, in the first place. Remember, pain is momentary but growth is necessary.

SELF-WORK

Putting in self-work requires 3 things: discipline, sacrifice, and assessment. These things are done in no particular order. I started with assessing what I was doing and thinking. Next, I started disciplining myself and lastly, I chose to start making sacrifices for my betterment. You can start with any of these, but they all must be done in synchrony. You cannot have more discipline without assessment and sacrifice. You cannot sacrifice more without discipline and assessment. Of course, without assessment, you wouldn't know it takes discipline to sacrifice. If one is willing to go on this journey, it can be one of the most agonizing things yet the most rewarding.

Putting in self-work is uncomfortably painful because it strips you down of your ego and then you are born anew. Call it a birthing or a rebirth, if you will. This is the true self, that carries its own truth and lives in its truth. If we take the time to go through this process, the pain becomes well worth the reward. We have been bred to be mindless in this system of illusion and it does not cultivate the truth within us. What happens is our egos get built up by our environment to help us make it in this world, but we become only fragments of ourselves. If we do not take the time to claim our true self, then no one will. Truth is in the soul of a person, our persona is nothing but a mask, a role we play to hide who we really are or want to be. Illusions of society suffocate the soul, forcing it into being what it is not. If we do not find our truth, then someone else will give us one. Let that sink in a bit. We came here to fully express ourselves and yet many of us simply exist. Most of us are distracted by everyday life and so we never take the time to go on that journey of Self-Work.

We deserve to be who we really want to be, but we must put in the effort to make our truth come to fruition. There will be times you will want to quit, doubt yourself, feel lonely, have withdrawals, and even want to turn back to what is familiar. The most important thing to remember is what you are doing it for. You are doing it to free yourself from mental captivity, programming, society, pretending, and to fully self-actualize.

THE FINISH LINE

How can I put this? There is no finish line! Somehow, we think that if we are able to just get to the end, there will be some type of celebration, fireworks and a medaling ceremony for us. That way of thinking sets us back because we try to map out what we have no control over and that is life in general. What we do have control over is our actions in life and even sometimes that can seem like a challenge. When the term 'finish line' comes to mind, we usually think of the final destination. Life is not linear; it is cycles that are continuous.

What we must master is how and what we do in those cycles. To think one day, you can just stop while in the middle of a cycle will only make you fall behind. The only way is forward, even when it's rough, confusing, or causing uncertainty to arise. If we never take the time to go our own way and discover our path, then we will run a race in search of an ending. But once you find your way you can make a path and once you make a path you leave an example for others who may consider going down it. A 'finish line' would imply that there is a race of some kind and a race would imply that there are placements of some kind. Everyone wants to know where they place or how they fare or do they stack up against the competition.

When you drive in your own lane, there is no competition. It's just you and the road ahead. When there is just a road ahead, it seems like you are free to go at your own pace and there is no pressure to be anywhere. Yet when others are on the road going different speeds, somehow, we feel the need to want to get around them or beat traffic just to get to a place we may not even want to be. That, my friends, is how the race goes! You win some, you lose some, and even when you win, you may not even think the rewards are worth it. Also, the 'finish line' can be moved by whoever is conducting the race and sometimes that may not be fair, but just think, you are choosing to participate willingly in this race.

When you remove the finish line, you remove the thought that it will be over soon. When you get over this thought of 'this is the only way I must win the race', you now open yourself up to endless possibilities. When you are willing to go through the cycles of life, you then remove limitations and find true freedom and growth.

SELF-EXPLORATION

When you are building this relationship with yourself it can be difficult to navigate. Just as it takes time to get to know people, when you are getting to know yourself on a deeper level that takes time too. Being a pioneer of your own internal world is not an easy task. You will encounter things that are fascinating about yourself and other things you can't stand about yourself. One thing to note is that without any exploration of your inner-verse (inside yourself), it will be hard to navigate the universe. The moment we begin exploring, it is exciting, and we want to know more. Well, when we tend to hit major roadblocks, we tend to want to quit exploring. Real explorers know that the journey may not be easy, but the journey of discovery makes it worth the risk. I cannot guarantee you comfort on this journey, but I can say that, if you go, you will be glad you did.

Navigation of the mind can be treacherous when dealing with unwanted thoughts and feelings. Make sure to take your time, remember this is not a race. It is you taking step by step action at your own pace. In order not to get lost in your own mind, you have to take the view of an observer. What I am saying is try not to be in it but look at it for what it is. Take for example when playing a sport, say soccer, while you are on the field as a player you can't see every action being made by each player while in play.

The only action you focus on are the actions you take. Now from a coach's perspective they tend to see the entire field, so they can see from a wider lens the plays the entire team is making. The coach would be the observer in the situation, while the player is actually in the situation. When in the mind, many thoughts and feelings can surface that can cause us to react as if we are a player in a game. If we learn the skill of observation, we can then choose the thoughts and feelings that best serve us in the long term. It takes time to learn this skill when dealing with the inner-verse. There are a vast number of things that can be uncovered there. Self-exploration we tend to overlook because it requires time that we think we don't have. However, when we walk our own path, we have all the time we need.

There is no one way to deal with the mind. That is why observing will allow you to see everything in front of you. When you are deep into something tunnel vision can occur, limiting one's vision. The best exploration is self-exploration because it will allow you to become keenly aware of behaviors, beliefs, thoughts, and feelings you never knew were there.

GETTING TO KNOW THE

DARK SIDE OF YOU

EVERYBODY HAS A DARK SIDE

Let me tell you something. If a person ever tells you they do not have a dark side, turn, and run for the hills. Reason being, either they aren't telling the truth, or they do not know they have one and the latter is more dangerous. If a person is not familiar with what they are capable of being or doing, then there is no telling of what they are capable of doing to you. Same goes if you are unaware. We all have this darkness inside and typically this is viewed as a bad thing but that is usually because this tool is used the wrong way.

Picture this. You are in the gym lifting weights and you work your way up to a weight that seems impossible to lift. Maybe you have tried to lift this on many occasions and you failed. One day you decide you are tired, pissed off, and you make up your mind that this weight will move by any means necessary. You are gritting your teeth, scowling at the weight, feeling this powerful sensation coming over you and you're pacing back and forth. Next, you go to pick up the weight and before you lift under your breath you say "it's going up". Then you scream, yell, breath vigorously and tense your entire body to finally complete the lift that has haunted you forever. After lifting the weight, you immediately drop it and get a dopamine rush from the accomplishment you just made. Finally, after so long of waiting, you get to say you have overcome. Now I am sure you wouldn't reach down into your sunshine bag of feelings to make this happen. When a predator attacks, no one smiles and says look, the predator is coming. You dig deep into the darkness to pull out that energy needed to bring it to the light. That is a healthy use of the darkness. When one is fully aware, they can go to that place and can control that darkness, it in turn does not get the chance to control them.

KNOW WHAT THAT DARKNESS IS AHEAD OF TIME

As discussed earlier, the worst thing is not being aware of your dark side and not knowing what you are capable of until a situation arises. The key to knowing this darkness is figuring out those parts of self that you may be embarrassed or ashamed of revealing. Learn this part of you and explore it. Why should you learn about the darkness inside? Well, let's talk about it. Have you ever had a time when you blew up over something that was so small you felt embarrassed afterward? Don't worry! If you have, you are not the only one. That was the darkness bubbling up inside and if you were aware then you could have controlled the output of that energy. Instead, it came out wild, loud, over the top, cruel and without substance. This is an emotional pull from the darkness, and it comes out without accomplishing nothing but making the situation worse.

When awareness of personal darkness is there, it can be filtered out, still get the point across and the message can be well received. Knowing this ahead of time allows for you to save yourself from fatal mistakes. Listen, the best communication is self-communication. If you only know one side of yourself then you are incomplete. When incomplete, one will never get the full benefit of being absolutely themselves. They will be something or somebody else in place of that incompleteness. The more you know ahead of time about yourself the better off you will be long term because you will be able to navigate better throughout life.

THE DARK SIDE CAN GET YOU THROUGH DARK TIMES

You may not know how right now, but what you are about to learn is how to use the darkness inside to push yourself toward betterment. Darkness is and has often been viewed as a negative thing. What may come as a shock to many is that the darkness always has its advantages. There is mystery in the darkness meaning there is something to be discovered while in a dark place. If we get comfortable in the dark, we then start to realize that this is just another part of ourselves that is untapped. Majority of what you read up until this point was how to overcome the darkness.

Now It is time to learn how to be comfortable in the darkness. In this place full of mystery, it can either be a place of strength or a place of failure. Nine times out of ten we look at our failure and let that be the determining factor. If we learn to understand before there is light there must be dark, we then come into a deeper understanding of first there is the unknown and then there is known.

Channeling is a valuable technique to learn how to deal with untapped darkness within oneself. This technique is used to take vast amounts of energy whether negative or positive and focus it into a singular action. The dark side of self is as real as the light side, but the key is knowing when and how to use it. When should this be used? Well, the short answer is in controlled spaces. For example, you are running and are trying to beat a qualifying time that you always seem to fall short on. You go through your same routine, put on your track gear, lace up your shoes, eat light, put on some upbeat music and head out. Every time you do this but to no avail because you never make the time you wish to achieve. Sometimes your skill or your talent is not enough. This is where you tap into something deeper - something more! You must bring out that deep emotion from the darkness into the light. That desire to go harder, practice longer, and run faster because deep down you know that time is within you to beat. The great separator is neither skill or talent. It is the character of oneself. In order to be the best version of self, one must go deep within the confines of his or her mind and bring that out. This means to know self, to the fullest extent. To know the dark and the light is to know the truth about who you are.

Once you know who you are (to a good degree), you don't have to hide yourself any more but you must continuously learn about yourself each day. There is no blueprint for this. There is only self-mastery and it is not an easy road. When you choose to go to these dark places, you will find ugliness, disgrace, sadness, hurt, and many other dreadful things. Guess what? They do not define who you are, so don't let it. Using those hidden sources of energy, you have just might be the push you need to hit that qualifying run time or build that strong character of a person whom you're striving to become. The state of "Knowing" is a choice, one can either choose to disregard certain aspects of self or know thyself.

Channeling dark energy is an art, and it can will a person to unbelievable heights as long as there is containment of the emotions that come along with channeling this energy. Getting to know yourself is like any other relationship. It takes time. It takes building trust. It takes concentrated effort. It takes vulnerability and it takes honesty. When a person has gone through these phases in a relationship, they tend to become good friends, close family or inseparable partners. This same process must happen within oneself.

No relationship can ever fully actualize until one goes through a process such as this one. The one thing to note here is that the majority of us go through this process with other people but not ourselves. Become who you are meant to be. The world is waiting on you but the world can't wait forever!

LOWER STATE OF MIND IS A

PLACE TO VISIT

NOT TO STAY

GO THERE

What are you waiting for????? Go! Stop making excuses! Go! Quit procrastinating and just Go already! Yeah, that's right go on go back to where you came, back to the darkness. You belong there anyway! Time out!! You may be thinking, 'Is this guy yelling at me right now? Well, no. I am using a few exclamation marks to get my point across. This is how I get your attention. Hey, I am attempting to lighten the reading or else you just might throw this book across the room and we can't have that. (Smile) All joking aside, the reality is you need to go to that empty space inside sometime. Yeah, it's no fun there because it is empty - like a house is not a home without furniture. But do you want to know the cool thing about an empty house? You can put in it whatever you want and come and go as you please because you own that shit.

Take ownership of your whole self and the deepest darkest recesses of your mind will become home before you know it. This can only be done through trial by fire. In order to pass a test, you have to first be tested right? Well, guess what life is going to do to you? Yeah, you guessed it. It will put you through some BS testing to see how you respond. The only way to get the upper hand is to study right. Going to that empty place in your mind may very well be the place you need to go to find newness or renewing of strength. Being empty means there is lots of room to be filled until full. Fulfill. Get it? Well, I tried. [Smile]The point is, when you go to places you have never been or have not been in a while, you have a higher capacity to learn something new. The more you learn, the more comfortable you become.

Being comfortable comes from knowing, knowing comes from experiencing and studying. Being afraid to go is understandable, and rightfully so, but not going means never learning and never learning means never becoming. The truth is, you can't afford not to go. Though these places inside the mind may not be what tickles your fancy, the truth awaits in those places. Never deny yourself the ability to learn, to build and to create. Every great thought or feeling you or any great person to ever walk this earth had has come from the darkness before it ever saw the light of day. You owe it to yourself to go and see what you are made of. Take some time for yourself to meditate, think and reflect. Now go to a tranquil place and begin your personal journey. It's time to start the process.

GET COMFORTABLE WITH THE UNCOMFORTABLE

Look who has finally arrived? Well, I hope you'll stay for a while. It has been a long time and it's time to catch up. This will be your consciousness talking to you, but the ego and base self are also present too. These 3 concepts represent the spiritual, mental and physical aspects of who you are. The question is which one is in control? When taking a trip to the dark, physical urges can arise, mental trappings are made evident and the consciousness is being tested.

The choice is simple - do you fall or do you rise up? As you stay on this journey, it will become clear as to what will need to be done but for now just try to get comfortable in the mess of it all. Normally, we want to hide from these thoughts or feelings but deep down we may want to act them out. Why not act them out in your mind, figure out if what you think or feel serves you or not. The greatest war is waged inside your head, but you can't win if you run from the enemy within. This is because it relentlessly keeps chasing until it corners you as its prey. Do not be a victim, you are a lion and, in order to exhibit bad-ass-ery, you must fight that inner enemy until it becomes your footstool and your prisoner.

COME BACK TO THE LIGHT

The darkness is never a place in which you want to stay. Remember you are just visiting. The point of going into the dark is to find something, but the point of coming back to the light is to reveal something. Never should the intent be to go to a dark place and stay so long that it becomes loathsome. You only want to go in with a purpose because if you wander into the dark aimlessly you may find more there than you are ready to handle at that point in time. Earlier, we spoke about how being in the dark space causes a feeling of being trapped, almost sucked in. This is why the intention must be to go in, find what you are looking for and get out - never let this place become your stomping grounds.

What the focus should always be is on discovery and channeling your energy into finding newness within you. Never forget to come back to the light because if you sit in the dark too long it will consume you and you will find yourself in that "dark space". It will be so subtle you won't even have the slightest clue of how you got there and why you stayed so long. There is another thing to note, when you go into the dark it is for yourself but when you come out to the light it is for others. Darkness is about reaching inward to the depths of oneself to pull out something the world has yet to see. If you come back to the light for selfish reasons, you are doing yourself and others a disservice. For the gifts that lie within us are meant to be shared with the outside world. Why don't you come back and show us what you have learned?

SHOW WHAT YOU'VE LEARNED

Time for show and tell. Let's see what you've got! Remember that in kindergarten all the kids brought in their favorite toy to share with the class. Well, that is what we do when we come back from the dark, we come back with stories, insight, experiences, truths and hopefully wisdom. We bring this to people in the external world to help move them and ourselves forward. I cannot stress this enough. We should get to know who we are on the inside, as well as how we are perceived on the outside. We often get caught up in how we are viewed outwardly but never ask ourselves who we are inwardly. This question is one that must be asked more often than not. If we are so caught up in the outer world, we will never learn anything new about ourselves besides what others perceive us to be. When this happens, our spirit becomes fragile because we do not know who we are. This is how depression, anger, confusion, bitterness, regret and so many other things start.

If you are not willing to learn about yourself then that means setting yourself up for someone to tell you who you are. Now, don't get me wrong. We should always seek wise counsel from people who mean right by us. They may see something we don't see that will make us better. However, we also must be able to stand our ground and the only way to do that is to know who you are and get around people who promote getting to know yourself. If you are lost, some people will take advantage of that instead of showing you the way. This is why it is imperative that you get to know the innermost parts of self so that you never become lost in the mind. When you are sound in self, you will exude confidence and people want to be around confident people. Interestingly enough, it sets the stage for what you will bring to show and tell.

People are interested or maybe even curious to see what you have learned. Some do not want to share because they may not feel confident enough to share. Guess what that means? You may have to go back into the dark to push yourself to discover more. When you push past the mental obstacles in your way, you will find confidence to come back and be open enough to share your truths. We all have to travel to very low depths in the mind to discover ourselves before we can reach the highest heights.

NEVER FORGET FROM WHENCE YOU CAME

Forgetting your failures and accomplishments lead to backtracking. For example: You left to go to the store, put everything in the shopping cart, piled it onto the conveyor belt, got up to the cashier and forgot your wallet. Yeah, that is what I mean! That sucks right? I mean you know you have the money but it's just not on you. You may feel a little embarrassed too, but you know you're good for it. The worst thing is that you wasted time, gas and brainpower to do it all again. There may have been times you did this and just said forget that I am not coming back because you were just over it. Well forgetting where you've come from in your journey can lead you to go astray or backwards.

The moment we feel we are fine we have this tendency to become oblivious to all of what we have experienced. Let me tell you something, I am guilty of this too. By no means do I have it all together. But why do we do this? My realization is that we have a natural aversion to pain. We do not want to feel that pain and the minute we come back to the light we forget the hell we just went through to get back. We come back and we don't share anything we have learned. We go back to the same things that lead us to ruin in the first place, then we make excuses, and fall back into negative thinking. Here we go again! Listen, as much as it may suck, own your pain, and don't become it! Remember, you cannot afford to forget. Keep your pain close and use it, don't let it use you! The minute you forget, that's equivalent to losing a part of you and now you have to backtrack to find that part again. Ask yourself do you really want to keep picking up the pieces? I know I just got passionate there but seriously there is no room for forgetfulness, when it comes to self-only mindfulness. Remember who you are and what you have become.

THIS IS PART OF YOU

NOT WHO YOU ARE

THE GOOD, THE BAD AND THE UGLY PARTS

Who said you had to be perfect all the time? The answer - society says so. We are never able to experience low points because if we do, we get demonized, criticized, or condemned for allowing ourselves to get into that position. We play as if things are alright on social media, social settings, family members and amongst our circle of friends. We, in society, tend to put up the front like it is okay but the reality is, it may not be and that is okay too. All parts of who we are may not always be the ideal or picture perfect. Having different aspects of who you are makes you human. The good parts of people we tend to admire, the bad parts of people we tend to inquire about and the ugly parts of people we do not desire at all.

Realistically, we are made up of all three. There cannot be one without the other but how we choose to deal with all parts makes all the difference. You are who you are, and you cannot change that. On the other hand, what you can choose to do is better who you are. It takes work. You may experience something bad and it may cause you to develop the ugly aspects of your character. Conversely, if you never have bad times and ugly moments you may never appreciate the good that can come from it. You may have heard the saying that bad things happen to good people well good things can happen for bad people too. The ugly side can come out of all of us and no one is exempt from that. Guess what? This side of us, though not the most pleasant, is necessary. It shows us where our character flaws are so that we can become more conscious of where we tend to fall short. To denounce or hide certain sides of you is to be untruthful to yourself and those around you. None of us came down here to earth with a manual for how to have great character, that must be developed through pressures of life.

To conceal who you really are for the sake of not being judged is to void yourself of the human experience. You are not here to please others just because it's the right thing to do. You are here to live your life and that means learning to ride the waves through the highs and lows of it. You have some character flaws; you have some quirks, and you have some admirable qualities. To be one dimensional is boring and stifles growth but to be multi-dimensional is to be free. Everyone loves the highs, but the learning is in the lows.

LEARN TO LOVE THE LOWS

What is there to learn during the low points in your life? Short answer, what you are made of. You have no clue of who you really are or what you are capable of until you experience some complications in life. These are teaching moments and there will never be a time to be more astute then, when you're going through something painful.

As a society, we tend to undervalue and underappreciate these moments but when it comes down to it these moments have made us either better or worse. Which one do you want to become? See, it's during the low points in your life where the work should be done. Will it suck? Yes, but will it be worth it? Absolutely! Instead of reacting during these times and getting emotionally involved causing you to further make undesirable choices, why not take the proactive approach? Meaning, take a few deep breaths, assess the situation and ask yourself what did I do that I could have done better? When you do this, it gives you back your power of control because who better to control you than yourself? Never put yourself in a position where you lose control over yourself! Side bar, there will be times when you lose control over yourself. It happens. It's a part of the learning experience in our journey throughout life. Does this make you a bad person because you lose control? No, it makes you an inexperienced person in dealing with certain emotions that may arise from unfortunate circumstances.

Expressing yourself is healthy and should be done. However, getting a handle on your state of being is another situation entirely. When you briefly lose your state of being you then are easily influenced by your external environment. Know this, you are only ruled by things you give power to. If you give power to the situation, it then takes rulership over your emotional, mental, and physical state. If I had a dollar for every time I lost control in the earlier stages of my life, I would have a nice little nest egg to sit on. In our youth, we are drawn to emotion like a moth to a flame and because of that we make choices that do not serve us well at times. This, though not necessarily enjoyable, teaches us more about how we conduct ourselves in a situation. From that point, we can choose to conduct ourselves differently or keep doing the same thing expecting different results.

Choosing to be in control is easy, when you have life going the way you want it. It is almost effortless, when things are going well. It is during low times where we are tested to see if we can remain in control of ourselves, when things around us are uncontrollable. The point is, you should always be aware of your state of being so that when your external environment is tampered with, your internal environment isn't shaken.

YOU AREN'T JUST ONE THING YOU'RE MANY THINGS IN ONE

You are capable of doing many things because you are many things. Do not box yourself in mentally because it will not allow you to express yourself fully. If you have a desire to reach certain goals in life, you will have to do something to reach those goals. If the goal is big enough, it will require some level of change on your part. A fighter, for example, may be pleasant to be around in social settings but in the ring he or she has to turn into a badass because 'it's do or die' for them in that environment. The fighter becomes a beast, in order not to become the prey. The fighter has to be assertive. If that fighter remains 'the socialite' in the ring, there is a good chance the fighter may get knocked down.

If a person wants to build a business but never had the experience of starting one, that person will have to go into another aspect of themselves to see that idea to fruition. That person may need to do market research, pay for coaching, create the right product or service, study their ideal clients' needs, figure out where to house their business and many other aspects. What if they have always been an employee? They will need to make the mindset shift, to acquire the knowledge necessary to become a business owner. You must always be in a state of becoming, if you want to see new realities unfold.

Have you ever had a time where you said, 'if I only would have done that sooner I would be where I want to be'? I am sure you have. We all have and that was because at that time we were not willing to become something else. That is because we limit ourselves in the way in which we think of ourselves. We definitively say "I am this" but never say "I could possibly be this as well". Why do we do that? It is because it is far easier to just identify with what is, what others

91

see us as and what we already know about ourselves. We restrict our capacity to go beyond that which is current. We prohibit the thoughts of something more once we figure out that it will require more from us. This is the 'comfort zone' and it deludes us into thinking things will always be like this. We even become fine with it especially if it is working in our favor. If we are satisfied with being the one thing we are at the moment, we may not even make an attempt to become something more than that.

Do yourself a favor right now and promise yourself that from this day forward you will be all things that you need to be in order to be all of who you are meant to be. Never sell yourself short of being all things you desire to be. There is a saying that goes 'the one is all and the all is mental.' This means you are a part of infinite consciousness and consciousness has no limitations.

WE ALL ARE BROKEN BUT THAT MAKES US HUMAN

You are so messed up but aren't we all? We tend to believe we are black sheep, when it comes to dealing with our own negativity but honestly everyone is dealing with sides of themselves, they wish didn't exist. There is not one person on the planet who has not dealt with a lower aspect of themselves that they didn't like, at some point in their life. It is a part of feeling alive when you feel the pain, the hurt and the grief but it does not have to define who you are.

No one has ever said 'I have it all figured out and I never have down moments or lows in life'. If they have, they are delusional. Some of us may have them more than others but we all have them. Experiencing the negatives in life actually brings us closer as a people. If nobody ever went through something, what would there be to teach? Would empathy ever be felt? Could commonalties be found amongst strangers? How would people know when it is time to make a shift in behavior? There is more to being in a negative state than we realize. We cannot always have it our way because that would make us closed minded by default. Negative energy can be used to kill the weaker aspects of ourselves to make room for new creation in ourselves and our lives. Negativity is an opportunity to correct flawed behavior or archaic ways of doing things. If we never encounter negativity, we would never have the chance to make a shift in our lives for the better.

You can't avoid all negativity in life but you can learn to use it as an empowering tool. Think about a scale from negative to positive. The further you go one side of the scale the more you are capable of going on the opposing side of the scale. Now let me explain, say the scale is numbered zero through ten. Five represents the middle ground, let's call that the gateway to the other side. Let's say that zero represents the lowest part of negativity and ten represents the highest part of positivity. If you have fallen to a two on the negative side, then you are capable of reaching an 8 on the positive side. In other words, the greater the pain on one side of the scale the greater the strength that can be reached on the opposing side of the scale. If you are going through something and there seems to be no way out of it, stop and think of strong people throughout history who have faced some of the greatest pains and turned them into some of the greatest triumphs the world has ever seen.

These people were not special in the sense that they were any different from you and me but the difference is they use their negative experiences to empower them in tough times. If they would have broken down, would we have witnessed great strides in people, societies and the world? Probably not. We all go through it; we all have flaws; we get lost in the darkness; we all are broken, but we all have the power to make a choice to pick up the broken pieces of us a 'head toward the light' within us.

DEAL WITH YOUR NEGATIVES AND NEVER STOP IMPROVING

Hey you! Why are you over there getting all emotional? Everybody goes through it. Why don't you just deal with it! Don't you hate when people say that to you? Certainly, it's not a favorite choice of words you want to hear in a time of being down. But is there some truth to this phrase? People who say "deal with it" are actually saying the right thing. They may just go about it the wrong way.

Listen, you can't control how someone may deliver the message to you but you can still choose to receive the message. If you were waiting for a special package to come in the mail, would you care how it got there? Would you care if the mail carrier put it in the mailbox or on your doorstep? As long as the goods you purchased weren't damaged inside, would you care how the box looked? Odds are that as long as it got to you and the contents within the package were fine, you probably would not care. Well, when someone tells us to deal with it, we may not like it at that time but they are correct in what they are saying.

We need to learn to be better equipped to handle and deal with negativity that comes our way. No one can do that better than you can. Trust me. It is not the easiest thing in the world but it is something that cannot be overlooked. What needs to happen is you must put the onus back on yourself. There is no way that you can get over something, if you do not take responsibility for your part in it. We tend to want someone or something else to take the blame, all of it. What happens here is by you putting it all on someone or something else, it disempowers you right away. It is almost to say that you were under the control of someone or something. Would you rather say you were being controlled or would you rather take responsibility? Both options are rough but the difference is responsibility comes from a place of being empowered.

Your negative self, energy and situation can be managed once responsibility is taken. Life has a funny way of showing us who we are and helping us dig deeper inside ourselves. We may shout at the top of our lungs, why me?!!! But what if we changed our perception by rephrasing the question into something like "you chose me?" or "is this for me?" Words are powerful, thoughts are too and so are our beliefs. When you take on responsibility, it then puts you back in the drivers' seat of your life.

You no longer are a victim of the negative position you are in, you become the owner of your position. That is a powerful move to switch your thoughts from 'why is this happening?' to 'this is meant to happen'. When you know something is meant to be then you can accept that shit! If we keep leaving our mess out there for someone else to pick up, it may be a long time before the floor gets wiped and cleaned, if you get where I'm coming from. Feeling down is one thing but never feel sorry for yourself.

You shouldn't want to wallow in sorrow over something you can possibly turn around sooner than later. Once you take responsibility and become empowered, take action. Start to work on your problem right away. One thing you can do to get over your down moments is to help someone in need who really needs it. It will make you feel more human and less like a monster or a 'scary cat'. Monsters have fears that no one sees them therefore they can't be validated, and 'scary cats' have fears that everything is after them and them only. To be an empowered human being means having the ability to set aside fear and make a choice of will it rule over you or will you rule over it. Remember, we as humans may not be the biggest creature in the jungle but our mind gives us access to infinite possibility. One possibility is the ability to overcome. Never stop chasing after what ignites the fire within you. Never stop striving for something more. The only thing in your way ultimately is yourself.

Everything else is a barrier and barriers can be broken. Improvement means going forward in a determined nature to show yourself and the world how much better you're working toward becoming something more. If we never work towards improvement, it means we are choosing stagnation. When in a stagnated state the spirit starts to die out of a person slowly and this can lead to, you guessed it, negativity. See, the purpose of this book is to help you feed the spirit again so that you can go back to leading the life you want to live. You can get back to chasing after what you feel is right for you or start to figure out what is right for you to go and chase.

Movement will get you to that "happy place" you want to be at but standing still will only magnify your lows and make you hesitant to take the next step in your life. You may trip and fall a few times along the way there, but it's better having scrapes and bruises in a place you want to be in than having no scars in a place you hate. Whatever you do, fail your way forward, you may take breaks to reset but never stop moving!!!

MAKING PEACE WITH YOUR

LOWER SELF

FORGIVE YOURSELF

Here comes the hardest part which is letting go of all the hurt, pain, misery, shame, and fear. It also comes down to forgiving yourself, others, and your past. This is not going to be easy and nor should it be. Forgiving takes place in the heart, and that is a really sensitive area. The heart has to be in a softened state to be able to welcome in forgiveness. Listen, you may never have expected to go through all of what you went through but the biggest thing any upstanding person can do is forgive. It takes a certain level of will to be able to do this. It is never easy admitting your faults or even calling out others on theirs, depending on what they mean to you.

Forgiveness is where healing can begin to take place in a person's soul. It does not mean to forget what happened to you. You may have gone through hell, so those memories shouldn't be cast aside. As brutal as they were, they were character building moments. If you let your heart harden, you will not reach that place of peace within yourself. It will always be someone, something or you causing you to fall into negativity. The only person who can stop that from happening is you. There is no room to hold grudges within when you are trying to break through into the realm of positivity. When you are down, start to practice forgiveness. A simple phrase like "I wronged you and I want to do right by you". Say this to yourself because once again this is you taking responsibility and ownership over yourself and how you choose to conduct yourself.

Start to question yourself by saying, 'what can I do to make things right?' 'What do I expect from others that I don't expect of myself?' 'Why am I still angry after all this time?' 'What is the real reason I feel this way?' 'What part did I play in all of this?' 'Why did I look to others for an apology when I didn't even ask myself for one?' Questions like these are thought provoking and not driven by emotional reaction but they allow you to proactively process your thoughts on the matter at hand. Having a deep internal dialogue with yourself will allow you to sort through your feelings, views, thought patterns, beliefs and give perspective. You may be thinking, isn't it crazy to talk to yourself? Well, if you believe it to be crazy, then it is. But let me ask you this, that voice in your head that is always talking isn't that you? No one is telling you to go around talking out loud asking and answering questions to yourself. Now that may be one who flew over the cuckoo's nest. (Smile)

Seriously, being in a quiet space with your thoughts can help you to discover a lot about yourself. Having that internal dialogue is a crucial part of being able to forgive. Forgiveness does not happen in the midst of noise. It happens in silence. When you are constantly being stimulated, you are not taking the time to quiet the mind and rationalize your thoughts. In order to forgive, you must listen clearly to yourself and that can't happen when everything is loud both in your head and in your surroundings. Be mindful so you can be fruitful. You can always return to the noisiness of the world but in silence you will find answers. When you forgive, you must forgive with all of your heart. What this means is you can't just say sorry and move on still with the lingering thoughts you had before you apologized. You have to be willing to empty your mind of all the garbage thoughts you had before, during and after forgiving. If you do not forgive, it will only hurt you and not anyone else.

Once you are willing to surrender your negative thoughts, emotions, and energy toward the matter at hand you then are ready to enter a state of forgiveness fully, without any anchoring to the past negativity. Furthermore, forgiveness is not just a one-time thing, there will be future moments in time where you will have to forgive so the more you stay in practice of it the easier it will become. Lastly, when you forgive, prepare for similar situations that may occur in the future so you won't find yourself forgiving the same things over and over again.

BUILD THAT RELATIONSHIP WITH SELF

The best ship you can be on is your ship so you can set sail on the course you would like to go. The best relationship to be in is the one with yourself, so you won't have to depend on others to fulfill all your needs but rather have those around who want to see your needs met. This is because they want to help, not because you put that responsibility squarely on them. If you are going to start relying on yourself, you are going to have to start building yourself. There is no building if there is no foundation. Who are you now? Who would you like to become and what do you see yourself doing? Have you asked yourself these questions yet? What about my gifts, talents, and skills? What comes natural to me? Why am I here and what am I supposed to do? Questions like this, help to set the building blocks for a good foundation.

Once the foundation is in place, you can build and mold your life on a solid ground. If there is no foundation in place, what you build will always be subject to falling down. Your relationship to yourself will determine how you interact with the world around you. If you are negative to yourself, you are bound to be negative to others and attract negativity toward yourself. I want to say before going further that the process of building oneself takes time just like building anything else. There are no shortcuts in this process, some things you will be able to move through quicker and other things you won't be able to move as quickly. This is alright because great things come in time. The self-building process goes as follows: foundation, blueprint and materials, framework, exterior and interior. Let's walk through what each of these stages represent:

- The foundation stage represents who you are at your core. In this stage you will lay the groundwork by asking yourself some tough, hard and thought-provoking questions. The more questions you ask the better. You can never not know enough about yourself. The more you know the better. If you ask the right questions, you may not like the answers you find but it will help you to problem solve sooner rather than later when the building process is underway. Doing this later will cause you to back track and who likes to do that. During this time, you will develop your core values and your WHY. Once you think you have a good idea of what you stand for and why you are willing to do what you must do then you should proceed to the next stage. By the way, none of this has to be perfect besides you always want to leave yourself open for change and growth.

- Next stage is the blueprint and materials stage. Here you will gather what you need to build out your character. This means books, audio books, podcasts, articles, coursework, study material, and keeping pen and paper around for note taking. This stage also represents what to focus on, what sacrifices should be made, what will be your disciplines, what knowledge will be acquired and how you will best spend your time.

- Following that stage is the one framework which represents how you see yourself living out life. What is the meaning behind the lifestyle you want to live? Why is it important to live this type of life for yourself? Here you must determine if you are being realistic with yourself or are you entertaining fantasy. Case and point - you may want to live life like 007. Now, who wouldn't but are you really going into espionage and working for MI6? Think about it. Anyway, this is where you cut the nonsense out and hammer down on what matters most to you as far as your needs and desires are concerned. This framework will house everything in it and protect from everything surrounding it. This life may be the only one we get so you might as well design the one you want while you are down here and live it out. If you think that you've managed to figure out the life you want to live and what it truly means to you, then let's move on to the next step.

- Next stage is the exterior. This stage represents how you want the world to see you. The people of this world will see you the way they want to see you because they are entitled to their opinions. However, the way in which you want to be pictured in the world is up to you. What do you want people to know about you? What do you want to be known for? What character traits do you want to display? Where do you want to live? Who do you want to be around? How will you transact with the world around you? These are all questions that will help you develop the external make-up of the lifestyle you wish to live out. When you have sat and thought about this a million times and have drawn the same conclusion multiple times, it's time for the final most difficult stage.

- Lastly, is the interior stage. This stage represents how you view the world from the inside out. If you view yourself as awkward, chances are you will come off a little awkward. If you view yourself as confident, chances are you will come off confident. Your interior is your personal thoughts, feelings, and beliefs about yourself. This stage is just as important as the first. The foundation stage determines what is vital to you living and why, but your interior stage determines how you will live out that which is vital to you. Simply put, your core foundation is the destination and your internal process is your compass.

These stages are subject to be altered throughout your life as you make achievements, grow, age, evolve, reflect, and strive for more. Once the building is built, you no longer have to start from the ground up; you can just make pivots in life when necessary. Worst case scenario, if your building falls for whatever reason then you already know how to rebuild again.

BECOMING WHOLE (LOVE YOURSELF)

Love is the greatest state of being to be in. This state of love comes from knowing oneself. If you never take the time to know who you are then how can you really say you love yourself. If you decide to be with someone else for love but you have not decided to love yourself, how will you know what love means to you? You won't be able to tell others how you would like to receive their love because you haven't taken the time to give yourself that. The reality is that you cannot be whole if you don't have love for yourself. The point of knowing how to deal with the negativity you may have or are currently experiencing is to know how to love on the parts of yourself that are less favorable.

If you can love yourself in times of negativity both internal and external, you can love yourself through anything. Becoming whole may be easier for some and harder for others, depending on the cards you were dealt. But in life it's how you play the hand you were given. Remember, cultivation leads to maturation, maturation leads to elevation and elevation leads to transformation. Become whole, become authentically you and become one with yourself.

FINAL THOUGHTS

My aim in this book was to open your eyes to some capacity about negative programming and how to overcome it. My intent was to provide you with insight on how to become and be your authentic self even through the darkest moments of your life. Every day is made new and some days will be greater than others but how we carry ourselves throughout that day and what we decide to do in it makes all the difference in the world. Let me tell you something, you were not meant to live your life for someone else, through someone else or beneath someone else. Your life is yours and yours alone but what you do with it can make the world move toward greater and better things.

Writing this book was very therapeutic for me as it allowed me to see how far I have come in my thought process and what a journey I have been on so far. This book was written because of the way I see how things are today. People are living low on hope, low on spirit and lacking knowledge about themselves. If we were able to tap into the power inside of us, we would understand that we have the ability to accomplish many things. There is a lot of hurt going on and that is because we have not been taught on a societal level how to deal with negativity and why it even exists. If we come to an understanding of what it is and what it means for mankind, then maybe we can begin to start major healing in the minds and hearts of many. I want those who have read this to know that no matter who you are, where you are from and what you have done, you are somebody and your life is worth more than you know. Do not ever get so lost in the dark that you don't find your way back because people around you are dependent on you and you are depending on you.

May your world be warm, may your future be bright, may your light shine through the darkest of nights.

Made in the USA
Las Vegas, NV
19 December 2021

38525217R00063